The Chapa Wellness Map

To God for all.

To my father, Francisco, and mother, Josefina, for their example and love.

To my family for their friendship.

To many friends and partners from the health, fitness, financial, and other industries worldwide, who have supported me in many ways all over the years. This new vision of the sports industry may benefit many; the world needs it.

And to all the people of the world who are physically active, my hope is that you enjoy reading this book to help you to keep having a longer and better life. For those who are not physically active, from the deepest of my heart, my desire is that you make yourself aware of the vital need to be more physically active and that you start moving today itself. All the effort, hours, and tiredness to write this book are worthy if just someone somewhere in the world is saved from death because he or she has started doing physical activity.

ORLANDO CHAPA

THE **CHAPA WELLNESS MAP** BE ACTIVE. BE WELL. BE ALIVE.

A Systematic Approach to Physical Activity

Meyer & Meyer Sport

British Library Cataloguing in Publication Data

A catalogue record for this book is available from the British Library

The Chapa Wellness Map

Maidenhead: Meyer & Meyer Sport (UK) Ltd., 2019

ISBN: 978-1-78255-158-4

Aachen, Auckland, Beirut, Cairo, Cape Town, Dubai, Hägendorf, Hong Kong, Indianapolis, Manila, New Delhi, Singapore, Sydney, Tehran, Vienna

 Member of the World Sports Publishers' Association (WSPA), www.w-s-p-a.org

Printed by Print Consult GmbH, Munich, Germany

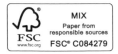

ISBN: 978-1-78255-158-4
Email: info@m-m-sports.com
www.m-m-sports.com

CONTENTS

PART I

PART II

PART III

PART IV

PREFACE

In October 2015, when I started visiting universities, organizations, and trade shows in Europe and the United States, looking for alliances to develop the required deeper research in the future of the topics analyzed in this book, I noticed that a complete book edition presenting the fundamental concepts of the project to explain in detail the general ideas and some practical applications of the *model* was necessary. In March 2016, a video was produced, which is now in YouTube as *World Wellness Network*, to present part of the project on an 8-minute spoken presentation; but this video is merely a very short overview of the whole idea. During the last two years, the content of the book has evolved to keep targeting the academic and scientific world, including access to entrepreneurs and people who do and who will exercise, so that many readers would benefit from the ideas, concepts, and tools presented here.

This book basically explains, from today's context, what is the *Chapa Wellness Map*, how it is developed, and how it could be used for any person—whether it is a father or a mother, personal trainer, CEO, club manager, entrepreneur, sports marketing strategist, physician, teacher, student, researcher, scientist, mathematician, software developer, inventor, economist, public policy maker, politician, human resources manager, insurance agent, businessman related to sports and fitness, and so on—to develop disruptive products, services, exercise techniques, studies, internet platforms, apps, gadgets, technologies, patents and, above all, to increase the quantity and quality of the life of any person interested in knowing where he or she is and where he or she should be in this classification system of the levels of wellness by physical activity. From there we can obtain the local, national, and the world levels, aiming to bring to an end the deaths caused by physical inactivity.

My hope is that you enjoy this first book and that you may be able to get, in one way or another, many benefits by reading it and applying the points presented therein and that many of you around the world would accept my sincere invitation to be part of this incredible journey seeking to get rid of our foe, *Physical Inactivity*.

ACKNOWLEDGMENTS

There are many people I have met in my life, from whom I have learned valuable things, for which I am very thankful. I believe that all those teachings have formed the way I think. Also, there are many people who have helped me and very much influenced my career as an entrepreneur and author that I am just going to write a list of the names without last names, but I know they will know who they are when they read this.

Francisco, Josefina, Diana, Francisco, Zovek, Octavio, Paty, Hilda, Irina, Mariana, Vincent, Diego, Alana, Zovek, Dara, Samuel, Estela, Magda, Marco, Anibal, Sergio, Octavio, Mike, Raúl, José, Miguel, Gabriel, Nicolás, Ralo, Roberto, Alejandro, Matilde, Gustavo, Katia, Brad, Julio, Luis, Catalina, Rolf, Eric, Salvador, Sergio, Alejandra, Daniel, Lourdes, Jorge, Hector, Elliot, Juan, Rodrigo, Oscar, Simón, Alfonso, Guillermo, Steve, David, Inga Lill, Arna, Ben, John, Erik, Luke, Host-Henning, Dameria, Sven, Daniel, Nick, Sue, Jeremy, Pablo, Jorge, Efrén, Robert, Eleazar, Helmut, Christine, Ludo, Marlies, Na Dine, Janez, Maja, Andrej, Robert, Victor, Terry, Jorge, Pablo, Daniel, Augusto, Claudia, Ángeles, Saúl, Javier, Héctor, David, Javier, Consuelo, Jesús, Malena, Manuel, Martin and many others, who, for sure, I am forgetting, but that does not mean their support has not been of great value for me.

Thank you, thank you very much for your friendship, teachings, and support; for those who are still alive, I hope we could keep constructing a better world together.

SPECIAL COLLABORATORS

Digitalization and retouch of original author's graphics made by Hot Marketing.
Front cover image made by Na Dine.
References systematization made by Consuelo Di Castro.

Thank you very much; great job!
—Orlando

INTRODUCTION

*In two atomic bomb explosions, about 140,000 people died in 1945;
can we generate a global chain reaction that could save millions
of lives every year caused by physical inactivity?—a World Wellness
Chain Reaction that brings and sustains life.*

—Orlando Chapa

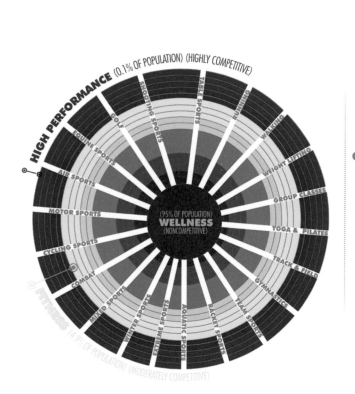

CHAPA WELLNESS MAP

A MODEL FOR SPORTS SUSTAINABILITY

"Sports promotion must converge to WELLNESS
and diverge to HIGH PERFORMANCE"

Orlando Chapa

CONTEXT

As we enter into the *Fourth Industrial Revolution*, with the use of Cyber-Physical Systems, the Internet of Things, the Internet of Services, Gene Edition, AI, Drones, and so on, in our daily lives, we face the contradiction that instead of having more time to take care of our health because of all this new technology, we have less physical activity at work and in our daily lives, with less time to workout because of many new digital activities that we do that are not physical, on one side, and, on the other side, we have more options for sport, training centers, training techniques, food, information, knowledge, and technology to improve and to track our workouts, bringing the paradox that approximately 3,000,000,000 people in the world are physically inactive with the negative result of increasing global problems related to this pandemic (diabetes, heart disease, cancer, obesity, etc.).

Last April 2018, I had the opportunity to visit the fair *Industry 4.0* in Hanover, Germany, the most important trade show in the world for the development of *Smart Factories*, a very important expression of the *Internet of Things*, where I was able to see the last innovations for automation and data exchange in manufacturing. *The Fourth Industrial Revolution* was first named here in 2011 in this fair as *Industry* 4.0. It was great to see a vast amount of technology altogether with all kind of robots, including some doing exercise; can you imagine that? It was funny and interesting; at least the robots don't get tired as we do. But until now, nobody and nothing can transfer all the benefits of doing physical activity into our bodies, so if we want to live better and longer, the daily required physical activity must be done by us.

In the middle of the exponential technology growth that we are starting to live, artificial intelligence (AI) and/or robots are defeating humans in many fields, and it is estimated by some tech commentators that by the year 2048, there will be AI or robots more intelligent than any human in general. They name it as a singularity, because this phenomenon has never happened before; around this trend, I just want to say that we humans have a *great asset in Physical Activity*, because until now robots don't need to exercise to function right (maybe in the future they may be manufactured with the necessity to be lubricated or to recharge their energy by doing some sort of robotic exercise . . . just kidding. Or predicting? So we have here this huge field as human right and as an opportunity to be less machines by doing physical activity or *Wellness* (as I redefined in this book), where we can get the best of our bodies by getting a great amount of benefits to feel, enjoy, and have a more and much better life, taking pleasure on the *Wellness of our bodies*.

For some futurists like Gerd Leonhard, *data is the new oil*, because of their economic, social, and political influence. *The Chapa Wellness Map model feeds on data*; therefore, we have a great opportunity for all technology developers to get involved in this model to help all the population of the world to know their levels of *Wellness by Physical Activity*, using the increasing options to obtain, process, and transfer the information related to the health of the body and connect all this *data* to the best options to improve and keep it.

Another interesting point that I want to comment to all the people involved in the *Fitness Industry* is that during 28 years in more than 80 trade shows in the 5 countries that I have visited, the winners of the Industry have been the equipment manufacturers. Life Fitness, Technogym, Precor Inc., Matrix, Cybex and others have done a great job in making state-of-the-art equipment by adding all the available technology to create great experiences for users, giving them the best workouts in a comfortable, safe, informed, and entertained way. However, we have some problem; the Fitness Centers, Clubs, Studios, and so on, have suffered to keep in business, and the leader Fitness Club brands of the 1990s were not the same as those of the 2000s—and these are not the ones that lead now. Why? Client's retention, price competition, and economy crisis are very hard to endure for almost all these clubs all over the world. But I hope that by applying some of the concepts and the model presented in this book, we would be able to help the clubs overcome this condition of the industry in some way. And let's remember that all the people involved not just in the health and fitness business but also in the sports industry in general face the challenge of having more than 5,000,000 deaths every year because of physical inactivity. So to all the CEOs, managers, businessmen, entrepreneurs, sports directors, personal trainers, teachers of group classes, coaches, and so forth, we have a great opportunity to create a new generation of disruptive business, institutions, products, services, and so on, to solve this situation in a sustainable manner.

Additionally, I have noticed another current situation—the fitness industry is too much focused on the fitness studios or fitness centers, and even though the current concept of *Wellness* keeps growing in these places with health-oriented programs, we have left a huge market unattended in some way (workplaces, schools, public spaces, houses, etc.); we have great opportunities for disruptive business in order to bring much better lives to many. It is my desire that many of you can grasp the concept of the *Wellness Model* presented here and that you apply it successfully.

This book, *Chapa Wellness Map*, has four main sections: (1) Presenting a New Model for Physical Activity (as an antithesis of the current model with its historical and economic impact on health), (2) a proposition for a World Classification System of the Levels of Wellness by Physical Activity (coming out of this new model or systematic), (3) the vision and the basis for the implementation (the formation of the NGO "World Wellness Network"), and (4) the applications of the model in the personal level (getting to know your current estimated level in the Chapa Wellness Map and to know where you should be) and in business (with the presentation of nonexistent business combining the Model and the technology of the fourth Industrial Revolution).

BOOK OBJECTIVES

The objectives of this book *Chapa Wellness Map: Be Active, Be Well, Be Alive—A Systematic Approach to Physical Activity* are:

Sedentary and Active People

a) That the *people* all over the world may be able to have a better understanding of the importance of integrating more physical activity into their daily lives and helping them to get involved doing it,

b) to know the technological trends that are bringing all kind of products and techniques to know more about the physical condition of their bodies and to exercise much better, and

c) to know that they can get a classification level that can help them to understand better where they are and to where they can go; in other words, they can get a number (to be more precise, a letter and a number) in a very fast and practical way that shows them where they should go according their own objectives and goals or at least to make them know where they should be so as to reduce the risk of diseases related to being inactive.

Instructors, Coaches, and Club Managers

a) That *Fitness Instructors, Sports Coaches, and Club Managers* may understand and apply the *Tools* presented here to give better teaching and service to their clients and pupils and that this new *Model* would help them to develop *innovative* and *disruptive* training techniques, products, facilities, camps, and so on;

b) by being in their work positions, more successful a virtuous growth cycle would be generated for the benefit of many, systematically activating the people of the world;

c) that the managers can diminish the *Attrition* percentage of the fitness studios and that a clear physical differentiation between a *Wellness Center* and a *Fitness Center* can be implemented by applying the new definitions stated here.

d) club owners and managers will notice that with more people getting active by using their facilities and coming out of the sedentary lifestyle, the clubs will be receiving more members looking for more specialized instruction and services.

Universities

a) That the *Universities* all over the globe would be able to not only integrate in their programs the *promotion of Physical Activity* for students, teachers, and workers but also generate more *research* of the costs, psychology, engineering, architecture, sustainability, geography, information technology, health, and so on, for a physically active society and for getting more understanding of the detailed damages of a physically inactive society;

b) that university researchers can develop *patents* in association with the university and private companies related to *Wellness*, generating wealth, and, above all, mitigating the problem of the world's extended sedentary lifestyle.

Hospitals

a) That *Hospitals* may have a new source to *encourage* patients to have a more active lifestyle as part of their preventive medicine programs and

b) that these *Health Centers* may get involved in *supporting* to do the assessments so that patients may know their current level in the classification system of the levels of wellness by physical activity explained in this book.

NGOs

a) That NGOs would find a partner at *World Wellness Network*, the NGO that will be formed to implement the basis that are going to be exposed in this book, to improve the levels of the quality of life of the world's population;

b) that more social entrepreneurs may get interested in creating new NGOs to work on the local, national, or global level, looking to finish with the deaths caused by physical inactivity.

Economists

a) That *Economists* all over the world recognize that Physical Activity and its Industry are important to achieve the *Sustainable Development Goals* of the *ONU*;

b)   and that to take the population of the world to a level where the risk of getting diseases related to physical inactivity can be considerably reduced, it is fundamental to improve the state of the world.

Businessmen

a)   That *Businessmen* related with Sports, Health and Fitness, and Physical Activity may be able to notice the *Population Segments* in the world that have been left with less attention;

b)   and to recognize that these segments are key for the present and future of the industry to take it to have a *bigger share of the Global GDP*;

c)   that *innovations* and *investment* can come to these new segments presented in this book so that people in need can be reached through the market; and

d)   that the *return of investment* of their business can be faster so that they can invest more, and, consequently, this industry can keep expanding, since this is a good industry that brings many benefits to the world.

e)   By using this model as a strategic management tool, they can anticipate rather than react to the disruptive technological and economic turmoil that we are living nowadays.

Technologists

a)   That Internet and App developers can find a *Disruptive* way to manage and display the information related to physical activity, fitness, wellness and sports;

b)   that new technology products, services, and experiences can be generated aiming to take to the *Wellness Sweet Spot* (see glossary)—the people of the world.

Politicians

a)   That *Politicians* could be more precise on their informs on this matter by reporting the *ranking* improvement of their nation in the world classification system in a very specific period of time;

b)   that they may be able to get supported by knowing other nations' *Good Practices* that will be available at the NGO *"World Wellness Network"*;

c)   that policy makers can develop better guidelines to create better cities and towns that can facilitate their populations to do physical activity; and

d)   that they recognize that physical activity gives *Health* and *Well-Being* to the people and that Health and Well-Being are a human right that was stated in the United Nations Assembly in Paris on December 10, 1948, when the *Universal Declaration of Human Rights* was proclaimed, specifically in the 25th article: (1): "Everyone has the right to a standard of living adequate for the health and well-being of himself and of his family...". Therefore, to make this right a reality in the lives of the people of the world and to bring to an end the deaths caused by Physical Inactivity, this concept of Physical Activity must become a global priority so that it must be added as a priority to Chapter 3 of the *Sustainable Development Goals* of the ONU.

PART I

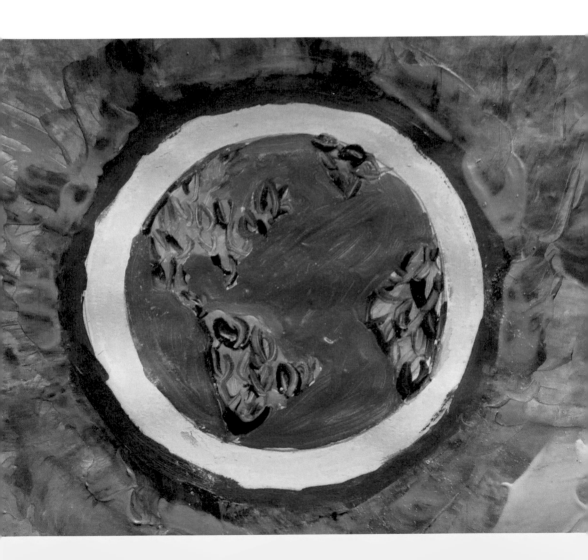

CHAPTER 1

THE COST OF PHYSICAL INACTIVITY

While the invisible hand looks after the private sector,
the invisible foot kicks the public sector to pieces.

—Herman E. Daly

THE COST OF PHYSICAL INACTIVITY

It is the 4th cause of death with 6% of total yearly global deaths.

Generates high cost to nations that are borne by tax payers, employers and individuals in the form of higher taxes.

In the USA, the Health Care Costs for Americans with Diabetes are 2.3 times (2.3 X) greater than those without Diabetes from data of the year 2017.

The United States assigns as an average $9,601.00 dollars a year on medical expenditures attributed to diabetes (2017).

The cost of Diabetes in the USA is staggering, $1 in $7 Health Care dollars are spent in treating diabetes and its complications (2017).

Alzheimer's effects won't be delayed by physical inactivity.

Physically inactive children do not attain better results at school.

18% of the total costs of this Pandemic are paid by the families.

10% Reduction in Global Physical Inactivity = Reduction of 533,000 deaths / year.

25% Reduction in Global Physical Inactivity = 1,300,000 deaths could be prevented.

Deadly as smoking

12% of depression and anxiety are attributable to physical inactivity.

In Northern Ireland 46%, Scotland 37% and in Wales 42% of adult population are physically inactive.

72.5% of German children and adolescents do not met the recommended levels of physical activity by the WHO.

In Russia economic burden of cardiovascular disease of €24,400.4 million (2009)

In developed countries has a cost of 1.5% to 3.0% of total direct health care costs.

It costs to the European Union (EU28) 80.4 billion Euros per year (2012)

Poland 2.2 billion Euros
Spain 6.6 billion Euros
France 9.5 billion Euros
Italy 12.1 billion Euros
UK 14.2 billion Euros
Germany 14.5 billion Euros
(2012)

In Israel overweight people spent 12.2% more than those with normal or below BMI ratio (BMI<25), 31.4% for obese people (30≤BMI<40), and 73.0% for severely obese people (BMI ≥40) 2010.

Physical Inactivity contributes to between 12% and 19% to the risks associated with the 5 major NCDS of China.

Cost of $6.8 billion Canadian dollars (2009)

In the US just 4% walk to work

The costs of obesity for the Aztec Country is of $6,000,000,000.00 dollars representing .6% of the Mexican GDP.

In Nigeria 41% of young adults (18 to 39 years old) Physically Inactive (2011)

In Brazil 220 000 life years could be gained with population overweight prevention programs

In Argentina Cost by cardiovascular diseases attributable to Physical Inactivity from 0.61% to 1.48% of the GDP (2017)

In South Africa 47% of adults live sedentary lives (2010)

Global pandemic

To the Australian economy is estimated to be $13.8 billion (2008).

31% Adults world wide (2.42 billion) and 4 out of 5 teens are not exercising enough.

Sedentary people have a 20% to 30% greater risk of heart disease and diabetes than regular excersicers.

Physical Inactivity cost to the global health care international system was of $53,800,000,000.00 dollars (conservatively, 2013).

16,178 Australians die prematurely each year due to physical inactivity (2008).

Not receiving the increase in mind concentration that excersite gives.

In 123 countries study shows that lack of exercise causes about:
6% of hearth disease
7% of type 2 diabetes
10% breast and colon cancers

"Physical Inactivity is costing us to many dead people"
Orlando Chapa

CONTEXT

Being physically inactive in modern times has been, for many societies, a symbol of freedom, development, and wealth—freedom because in the past, in some regions, heavy work was done by slaves, so free people were more inactive related to work; development because many industrialized countries have utilized more mechanized systems, compared to those countries that are not, into their productivity chains, allowing many of their habitants to be more physically inactive; and wealth because in some societies wealthy people hire lower-income people to do the heavy physical work that they do not wish to do.

However, since the last decades of the 20th century and as an increasing trend in this 21st century, the perception and need to activate people worldwide has been growing intensely, and the fundamental reason of this is *Health.* Today, *the Cost of Health* caused by Physical Inactivity is attracting an increasing attention to Global Institutions, National Governments, Corporations, Insurance Companies, Managers, Families, Instructors, and Individuals, because it is high in economic terms and in the quality of life that is lost.

COSTS

Costs to Individuals

Today, it is becoming well known that physical inactivity causes diabetes, and this disease brings many complications that diminish the quality of life of the one who has the disease; problems would be with the heart, eyes, kidneys, nerves, foot, skin, teeth, and other parts of the body. Just to exemplify, in the United States, from data collected in 2017, the health care costs for Americans with diabetes are 2.3 times greater than those without diabetes. In this study, it has also been calculated that a person in the United States assigns as an average $9,601.00 dollars a year on medical expenditures attributed to diabetes. This is a very high cost that many people have to pay because of lack of exercise and an unhealthy diet. And we are talking just about the effects of the diabetes; physical inactivity is associated also with heart disease, osteoarthritis, breast and colon cancers, depression, and anxiety among others. In October 2015, I had gone to visit my brother in North Carolina, United States; he received two phone calls in a week from his health insurance company inviting him to reduce his corporal weight, offering a discount on his monthly fee by reaching the goals established in a program that they had made for him. This is just an example about the savings any person can get by being *Physically* more *Active*.

In Israel, a study by Gary M. Ginsberg and Elliot Rosenberg, with data of 2010, published by the *Israel Journal of Health Policy Research*, presents that overweight people spend 12.2 percent more than those with normal or below BMI (Body Mass Index, see Glossary) ratio (BMI<25); the percentage was higher (31.4%) for obese people (30≤BMI<40) and even higher (73.0%) for severely obese people (BMI≥40).

Costs to Families

Physical inactivity is as deadly as smoking and generates 10 percent of premature deaths. Besides all the monetary costs to families that being sick generates to them, the economical and emotional effects that a premature death brings to families are almost catastrophic, which are created just because of the bad habit of not doing exercise and not having a good diet. A dysfunctional family will be generated, who will reduce, in many ways, the well-being of their members, and the possibility of better aspirations of the younger members will be reduced because of the lack of leadership, support, and income that the deceased will not be giving to the family.

Doing some calculations, from a study published by *The Lancet* in 2013, due to being physically inactive, $9,700,000,000 dollars are spent on health care costs in most households. If we divide this number by $53,800,000,000 (conservative total global expenses on related health care costs), we get that the family pays 18 percent of the total cost of this pandemic.

Costs to Corporations

Absenteeism has a high cost, but *Presenteeism* (at work; but out of it, it can be more correctly defined as productivity loss resulting from health problems) has a higher impact in the productivity of workers, thereby incurring more costs to the companies. Just imagine people at work who have type 2 diabetes who feel bad or tired because their physical strength is diminishing. The problem is hidden because the worker is physically present, but how he or she feels is something we don't exactly know, and this affects his or her performance and his or her happiness at work. It has been calculated by researchers that Presenteeism can reduce the productivity of an individual by one-third or more. As an example, in the United States, in 2017, the cost of diagnosed diabetes related to reduced productivity was calculated to be $90,000,000,000 dollars.

It has been published by *The Lancet* in the United Kingdom that in 2013, $12,900,000,000 was the total expenditure by the private sector toward costs generated due to physical inactivity all over the globe, and this number represented almost 24 percent of all the costs together: households, public sector, and private sector.

Also, companies have to pay higher life-insurance premiums for obese employees than for those who are not. Physically inactive workers concentrate less on work than those who exercise regularly; people who feel better at work because of their physically active lifestyle are more productive for their companies. In the spring of 2016, I visited the headquarters of some Silicon Valley companies such as Facebook, Google, and Apple and found that they intensely promote the use of bicycle to get to work; all of them have workout stations, with the latest training techniques and equipment, because they are convinced that it is good to invest in the development of *Corporate Wellness* so as to diminish the cost of physical inactivity at work. The *Chapa Wellness Map* definitively can help to activate people at workplace by helping them to know, in an easy and fast way, what is their *Wellness Level* (as defined in this book) and to show them where they should go. We have already talked with the publisher to write a second book focused on this important task in order to change the mind-set and environment of the companies and to support them to get healthier, happier, and more productive workers.

National Costs

All over the world, the governments of countries like Slovenia, Holland, Canada, Mexico, Germany, the United States, the United Kingdom, Australia, China, Brazil, South Africa, Nigeria, among others, have realized that a physically inactive population costs too much money to their national health systems and that those problems would be solved by increasing the attention to the causes and investing resources in prevention rather than in correction. The intention of this book is to propose a solution by creating a systematic approach for physical activity (Chapa Wellness Map), giving the basis for the *World Classification System of the Levels of Wellness by Physical Activity* that will be used in the *NGO World Wellness Network* to implement the system and to share good practices with all the nations in the globe.

For example, the cost of diabetes in the United States is staggering, as published by American Diabetes Association on March 22, 2018, where the total cost of diagnosed diabetes has risen to $327,000,000,000 in 2017 from $245,000,000,000 in 2012; this represents an increase of 26 percent in that period. In 2017, more than 30,000,000 Americans had diabetes, and 84,000,000 had pre-diabetes; out of $7 spent for overall health care, $1 was spent in treating diabetes and its complications.

Also, $31,200,000,000 were paid by the public sector in 2017, representing almost 58 percent of the total of international expenditures in physical-inactivity health care costs, where we can see the burden faced by the governments of the nations because of the lack of a new model on the sports industry that would have actually helped in solving this global pandemic.

On the Physical Inactivity and Sedentary Behavior Report of 2017, published by the British Heart Foundation, we found that around 20 million adults in the United Kingdom are physically inactive; 39 percent of adults in the United Kingdom do not meet physical activity recommendations; heart and coronary disease cause over a quarter of all deaths in the United Kingdom; in Northern Ireland 46 percent, in Scotland 37 percent, and in Wales 42 percent of adult population are physically inactive, and that around 60 percent of adults in the United Kingdom are unaware of the Government's physical activity guidelines.

On Medibank's 2008 report of the Cost of Physical Inactivity, we can read that the cost of physical inactivity to the Australian economy was estimated to be $13.8 billion, and it was estimated that 16,178 Australians die prematurely each year due to physical inactivity. Also, the direct health cost attributable to physical inactivity in millions per year in 2007–2008 was $399 for coronary heart disease (25%), $174 for stroke (11%), $226 for type 2 diabetes (14%), $45 for breast cancer (3%), $66 for colon cancer (4%), $190 for depression symptoms (12%), and $503 for falls (31%); this gives us a total of $1,603 million of the total gross cost of physical inactivity. In a very interesting accounting of the physical activity economy, they estimated that the direct cost of being physically active (sports injuries and fitness-related expenses) was a total of $884 million, so we have $1,603–$884 = $719 million per year as an estimated Net Cost of Physical Inactivity. Very interesting numbers!

Germany adopted the World Health Organization's Global Recommendations on Physical Activity for Health (2010) as its national recommendations, and from the Germany Physical Activity Factsheet of the EURO WHO, we come to know that between the years 2003 and 2006, German children and adolescents (3–17 years), of which 29.4 percent are males and 25.4 percent are females, having an average of 27.5 percent, reached the recommended physical activity levels of the WHO; here we can easily see that 72.5 percent of German children and adolescents did not meet the recommended levels of physical activity.

The Mexican government has been investing hard, installing exercise machines in public spaces all over the country, and has been promoting on the media a very good program, orchestrated by the Ministry of Health (Secretaría de Salud), which aims to help people check their weight, reduce calorie intake, and move (*chécate, mídete, muévete*), due to the alarming levels of overweight and obesity in all segments of the population and the very high burden of economic costs for the public sector that this situation generates. A March 17, 2016, report of the CONACYT (the public science and technology organism of Mexico), from a study made by two universities—UAM and UNAM—estimated that the economic cost of obesity for the Aztec Country was $6,000,000,000 US dollars. This quantity represents around 0.6 percent of the Mexican GDP; that is, about the same economic size of the expenses in Mexican Science or in Mexican Military or in the total Sports Mexican Industry.

In Canada, the total cost of physical inactivity in adults in the year of 2009 was $6.8 billion Canadian dollars, representing 3.8 percent of the overall health care costs, in a study made by Ian Janssen (Associate Professor and Canada Research Chair in Physical Activity and Obesity, Queen's University, Canada).

In a study realized in Argentina, published in 2017 by "Revista Panamericana de Salud Pública 41, e92), it was reported that the economic cost for cardiovascular diseases attributable to physical inactivity were from 0.61 percent in the minimal scenario to 1.48 percent in the maximum scenario of the GDP.

In Brazil, in a report presented in the OECD page "Third Lancet Series on Chronic Diseases: Brazil-Key Facts," almost one in two men and over one in two women are overweight. Here I have found an interesting prevention approach; it says that "up to 220 000 life years could be gained through a combination of prevention programmes in Brazil every year."

In China, we have similar results, but having 1,415,045,928 habitants (2018), any cost will impact in an important manner the whole world numbers. On this study, published in November 2012 in ResearchGate by Juan Zhang (Peking Union Medical University) and by Jad Chaaban (American University of Beirut), the total economic burden of physical inactivity in China has been estimated; they obtained it by combining the medical and nonmedical costs of five major non-communicable diseases (NCDs) associated with inactivity, and some of the most important results were that "Physical Inactivity contributes to between 12 percent and 19 percent to the risks associated with the 5 major NCDs of China, namely, coronary heart disease, stroke, hypertension, cancer and type 2 diabetes. Physical inactivity is imposing a substantial economic burden in the country, as it is responsible alone for more than 15 percent of the medical and nonmedical yearly costs of the main NCDs in the country."

In South Africa, with data of 2010, 47 percent of adults lived sedentary lives, more than double the global average that was 23 percent in that year; more than 60 percent of Colombian and Saudi Arabian adults fall in this category as well.

In Nigeria, a study published in 2011 reported that 41 percent of young adults (16 to 39 years old) were physically inactive, women being more likely to be inactive than men.

In the Russian Federation, the cardiovascular disease is the first cause of death, with an economic burden being € 24,400.4 million in 2009, with 21.3 percent due to health care and 78.7 percent due to non—health care costs.

Global Costs

According to the WHO, physical inactivity is a *Global Pandemic* today, which is the fourth leading risk factor for global mortality, 6 percent of global deaths, causing more than 3.2 million deaths every year globally. Moreover, physical inactivity is estimated to be the main cause for approximately 21–25 percent of breast and colon cancers, 27 percent of diabetes, and approximately 30 percent of ischemic heart-disease burden, and so on. According to the WHO, "Physical Activity is defined as any bodily movement produced by skeletal muscles that requires energy expenditure" and that "Regular moderate intensity physical activity—such as walking, cycling, or participating in sports—has significant benefits for health. For instance, it can reduce the risk of cardiovascular diseases, diabetes, colon cancer, breast cancer and depression. Besides, adequate levels of physical activity will decrease the risk of a hip or vertebral fracture and help control weight." More than 3.2 million deaths occur every year, and according to some other reports, this number has increased to more than 6 million in the same period of time. I believe that we have a war to fight here, and the enemy—"Physical Inactivity"—has been fighting worldwide with success; we need research from all over the world to be more precise to know the global, national, and local costs of this pandemic even to the point to know the family and personal costs of Physical Inactivity. These are some of the aims of the NGO that will be formed: *World Wellness Network* and other entrepreneurial activities that we will be promoting.

The Lancet, by doing some personal comparisons, has published a study that shows that the estimated conservative cost of physical inactivity to the global health care international system was $53,800,000,000 in 2013, results that is close to the total GDP of Bulgaria in the same year and similar to the total revenue of Intel Corporation, which was also the 54th largest company of the world in that year.

And, finally, I want to share with you a very interesting concept—the DALY. The WHO defines it thus: "One DALY can be thought of as one lost year of 'healthy' life. The sum of these DALYs across the population, or the burden of disease, can be thought of as a measurement of the gap between current health status and an ideal health situation where the entire population lives to an advanced age, free of disease and disability." Using this concept, we, in the same study of 2013 published by *The Lancet*, understand that Physical Inactivity was responsible for 13.4 million DALYs worldwide.

We are losing too much *Wellness* all over the world, don't you think?

CHAPTER 2

PHYSICAL ACTIVITY THROUGH TIME: LABOR – SPORTS – PHYSICAL CONDITION

*Seems that our bodies do not forget that they
need to do physical activity to have Wellness,
because for thousands of years it was necessary to survive.*

—Orlando Chapa

CHAPA WELLNESS MAP

PHYSICAL ACTIVITY THROUGH TIME
LABOR - SPORTS - PHYSICAL CONDITION

YEAR	?	-10000	-7500	-3500	-1200	-600	500	1500	1760	1860	1940	2011
AÑO	?	PALEOLITHIC -10000	MESOLITHIC -7500	NEOLITHIC -3500	BRONZE AGE -1200	IRON AGE -600	CLASSICAL ANTIQUITY 500	MIDDLE AGE 1500	EARLY MODERN ERA 1760	FIRST INDUSTRIAL REVOLUTION 1860	SECOND INDUSTRIAL REVOLUTION 1940	THIRD INDUSTRIAL REVOLUTION 2011	FOURTH INDUSTRIAL REVOLUTION

LABOR, **SPORTS**, **PHYSICAL CONDITION**

YEAR	?	-10000	-7500	-3500	-1200	-600	500	1500	1760	1860	1940	2011
AÑO	?	PALEOLITHIC -10000	MESOLITHIC -7500	NEOLITHIC -3500	BRONZE AGE -1200	IRON AGE -600	CLASSICAL ANTIQUITY 500	MIDDLE AGE 1500	EARLY MODERN ERA 1760	FIRST INDUSTRIAL REVOLUTION 1860	SECOND INDUSTRIAL REVOLUTION 1940	THE DIGITAL REVOLUTION 2011	INDUSTRY 4.0

LABOR, SPORTS, AND PHYSICAL CONDITION

From hunting, fighting to survive, and natural harvesting from plants and trees to the use of drones, the Internet of Things, AI, and cyber-physical systems, humanity has been giving a *Long Jump* into modernity, causing a shock in our bodies, without giving them enough time to adapt to these new conditions; they are complaining, as if they are screaming, "Here we are! Help us; we need to move . . .!"

In this chapter, I will compare 12 time periods of human history with three segments of human physical activity—labor, sports, and physical condition—looking for a better understanding of our current situation on this matter. I did it in this manner because these three concepts have been and remain intrinsically correlated through all human existence. (Some may say that any kind of sport, as we have defined in history, has not been practiced by humans since the beginning of its existence. I do not have any proof for a yes or a no at this point, but by logic at least we could say that labor and living have always given a specific state or condition to the human body, even though this was not measured until recent years.) Further, these three concepts are important to grasp the *new definition of Wellness* that I am presenting in this book for a *new Model* for the sports, fitness, wellness, and physical activity industry.

This chapter is not looking to be an exhaustive collection of research in human history; I just want to present some contextualization for the main topic that I am analyzing in this book—that is, how we can live better and longer through a more sustainable model for physical activity, because of the current crisis that in this matter we are all living nowadays.

Paleolithic Age

Known as the Old Stone Age as well, we are talking about more than 12,000 years in the past; some authors comment that it "ranges from the first known tool use roughly 2.6 million years ago to the end of the last Ice Age 12,000 years ago," where we can see that heavy physical activity was fundamental for surviving and that the first sports were a simulation of real working-life situations, such as wrestling and sprinting. For our modern mindset, it is not easy to grasp, at least for me, how a group of "business partners" in the Paleolithic age could have gone out there to kill a mammoth to get the protein supply of the season for their families, or how using stones as tools may have been the most advanced Industrial Technology of the time; but analyzing these facts, from modern perspective, the overall physical condition of the population was good, because physical activity was intense almost for everybody, even though the life-span was short because of many other reasons not related to physical inactivity. Casually, this morning, while I was hiking on a small mountain, I took two small stones to add some weight while walking; I can say that unconsciously I was getting into the Stone Age mood.

Mesolithic Age (10,000 BC–7,500 BC)

During this era, also called Middle Stone Age, the ice that was on the earth slowly melted. The domestication of plants and animals began, hunting started to decline, and the use of more stones as tools appeared, so they had a new way to get strength and mobility just by doing the daily work; they were mostly physically Fit. Diet started to change because of the milk produced by animals and the production of plants by the emerging agriculture. Archery also appeared around 9,000 BC, along with fishing, to survive; to practice for the real-life situations may have been a good sport. We could compare this *imitation* of real-life situations with today's *functional training* that many coaches and instructors seek in order to prepare today's people for the daily physical demands of our time.

Neolithic Age (7,500 BC–3,500 BC)

This period is also referred to as the New Stone Age. In this era, cereal production started, and new crafts and the division of labor appeared such that new natural workouts requiring different muscles and skills were built, and heavy physical activity was prominent for almost everybody; even though people started to live in villages, meaning they were not being nomads anymore. An important element was introduced into the human diet that has been related to our health since that time; this was the introduction of alcohol in the form of fermented fruit. The invention of the wheel in the late Neolithic Age was an important game changer in Labor and Physical Activity. Swimming started, and working out became more diverse. We find that religion appeared soon after, with worship to gods, so I think this was a proof of some kind of meditation or mindfulness that started to give humans a more balanced *"Neolithic Wellness"*

Bronze Age (3,500 BC–1,200 BC)

This was a period where the extensive use of metals began, and many new workouts were developed while working every day. But then the context changed, and human progress slowly started to accelerate. Boats were used for transportation, powered by humans; new muscles and training were involved. Mesoamerican ball game appeared and then shooting and different kinds of ball games in Egypt were practiced. The proliferation of the use of scales by merchants grew, and these scales were the foundation of the ones that we use today to check our weight. Moreover, in this age, scales were built. The entire population was very active.

Corporal analysis and assessments are key today to defeat Physical Inactivity, and to start measuring our body, it is also important to have technology.

Iron Age (1,200 BC–600 BC)

In this age, the use of steel grew; people noticed that iron was stronger when carbon was introduced after being left in coal furnaces. Tools and weapons were made out of iron or steel; blacksmiths appeared, and their bodies could be a good example of the physical condition of many workers during this time. Farming was easier, but it still needed hard physical effort. The first Olympic Games were organized in Greece in 776 BC, so we could also say that the foundations of our modern sport system started here. Can you imagine? All the records to be broken in Olympic Games in the future, all the national gold-medal champions, and national Olympic heroes who would come. Our present sports model was settled here in the Iron Age, where I can say that iron athletes emerged to make history while High-Performance level in sports started to be developed. Chariot racing, dancing, and pentathlon were practiced as sports in Greece in this time as well.

Classical Antiquity (600 BC–AD 500)

This was a period of Homer's poetry, the emergence of Christianity, and the decline of the Roman Empire. Slavery was notorious in Greece and Rome, so, for many, heavy physical activity to survive was by force, without any freedom, and for some it was diminish in an important manner. The Olympic Games were celebrated every four years since 776 BC until AD 393 in Greece, and they were not organized again until the 19th century. In Rome, gladiators—strong men fighting for their lives—performed a very special spectacle those days, portraying many physical and combat skills. I want to make a comparison that could be applied in our days; the Greeks were more oriented to health, image, and competitive physical activities, while the Romans were more oriented to military, displaying physical strength and abilities for combat. So, in a nutshell, the Greeks were more oriented to *Wellness/Fitness/High-Performance* activities, while the Romans were more oriented to *Fitness/High-Performance*. The Greeks and Romans used calipers for measuring; in our days we use a special type of Caliper to measure Body Fat Percentage, an important measurement to know our level of physical condition.

Middle Ages (AD 500–AD 1,500)

From the collapse of the Roman Civilization to the Renaissance, this was a period of migration. Agriculture was very important, the use of the plough facilitated the work, but this was physically demanding for the people in the fields; long-distance navigation was predominant (America was discovered), and, in general, heavy physical activity was required for most of the people to live. New sports were developed, such as medieval football, calcio fiorentino, fencing, and horse racing. In Northern Europe, barbarian tribes needed good physical condition for survival, because being physically strong for war and the skilled use of the sword were two very important aspects. Because of theological beliefs, the body was seen as sinful, and in a few cases that remains the same in some religions today, even to the point that some people even believe that exercising is not required to please God; a religious reform is required, at least in some aspects. Chess also was played in this time, and mind training started to evolve (concentration, strategy, and patience).

Early Modern Era (AD 1,500–AD 1,760)

This was a period of globalization, where Renaissance and Enlightenment came, the scientific revolution and age of reason began, and Copernicanism rose. (I want to make a comment here: In the global sports industry today, I believe we must make a shift in thinking, to put in the center of a new model the fundamental segment of the population in order to solve the pandemic of physical inactivity that we have nowadays, just as in those days when they made the Copernican Revolution). Great Britain had a great increase in agricultural productivity, mercantilism, and international trade, but heavy physical activity at the workplace was needed for the majority of the population to live, yet. AD 1660 marks the origin of professional sport (cricket in England). Cricket, horse racing, and boxing were financed by gambling interests (England). In 1553, the Spaniard Cristobal Mendez published the first book that addressed exercise and its benefits (*el libro: Ejercicio Corporal y sus Beneficios*), where he gives a medical viewpoint regarding sports and physical activity. Martin Luther and John Locke espoused the theory that good physical condition enhanced intellectual learning. So we are moving to the beginning of the technological revolutions that changed dramatically the way we work and live, and our bodies testify to this.

First Industrial Revolution (AD 1,760–AD 1,860)

The mechanization of production using water and steam power marked the revolution that began to reduce considerably the heavy physical activity at the workplace, which existed through all human existence, but now long labor schedules are hard for many people. We have here an important shift from an agrarian to an industrial economy; I see here an important transformation at the workplace that has damaged our health: in the agricultural production fields, people were around nature for many hours, enjoying free landscape, oxygen, sun, soil, plants, moving, and so on, but after being transferred inside these new factories, it was, and still is, hard for many. But, in general, the standard of living of the population began to increase due to the growth of income, and GDP per capita started to grow, even though physical inactivity began to emerge for many with nonstop until today. Population also started to grow in a remarkable manner. In England, universities started to compete with one another in sports. Baseball came into existence and appears to have evolved along with cricket. With the leisure that the First Industrial Revolution developed for some people, more players and observers of sports were generated. Physical education programs expanded within the European nations. Exercise facilities called TURNVEREINS or TURNPLATZ were built in Germany for running, jumping, balancing, and climbing; they were developed by Friedrich Ludwig Jahn starting in 1811. Benjamin Franklin in the United States widely recommended physical activity.

Second Industrial Revolution (AD 1,860–AD 1,940)

This was a period where mass production was introduced with the help of electric power and line production. In 1870, the work done by steam engines exceeded that done by animal and human power, thereby greatly reducing the hard physical work required in some factories. But in many nations, this did not happen, as living in the cities required less physical activity. In 1894, Baron Pierre de Coubertin founded the International Olympic Committee (IOC). In 1896, the first Summer Olympic Games (modern era) were held in Athens, Greece. In 1924, the first Winter Olympic Games were held in Chamonix, France. Tennis Davis Cup started in 1900 as a competition between the United States and Great Britain (in 2018, 132 nations are involved). In 1903, the first World Series were played in the United States. In 1930, the first FIFA World Cup was played in Uruguay. In 1870, Adolphe Quetelet published a book on anthropometry, where he proposed the *Body Mass Index (Quetelet Index),* which is key today for our assessments. In 1881, Samuel Siegfried Karl von Basch invented the blood pressure meter.

Thus, we see that with the help of all these new technologies, new methods were developed to measure the progress of physical condition. President Theodore Roosevelt, taking himself as an example, encouraged the US population to indulge in physical activity. We are now having in a mature state the labor, sports, and physical condition that has prevailed in our lifetime, and the next two industrial revolutions would come, bringing an awesome future for everybody. We must take a look into the future, to see what will come in the Sports Industry; to see how we can start to redefine *Fitness* and *Wellness* today; this is my heart and this is a *Core* theme in this book

Third Industrial Revolution (1940–2011)

This period is also called the Digital Revolution. Shifting from mechanical and analog electronic technology to digital electronics, computing and communications technology expanded greatly with the Internet and the smartphone. The Digital Revolution marked the beginning of the Information Age. The bases for a more inactive lifestyle were established here because unlike before, physical activity at work wasn't required to make our everyday living. This Digital Revolution was terrible for the physical condition of kids because of video games kept them physically inactive; however, the kids have obtained other good skills and entertainment. In 1946, Formula 1 was defined with the FIA standardization of rules. In 1948, the first international Wheelchair Games were realized. In 1950, the Ladies Professional Golf Association was founded, and in January 1967, the first NFL Super Bowl was played in the United States. In July 1969, man walked on the moon. In 1970, the first New York City Marathon was held. In 1983, the first World Championships in Athletics were realized. In 1995, the Extreme Games were founded. In 1947, Dr. Thomas K. Cureton introduced testing for cardiorespiratory endurance, muscular strength, and flexibility. The *modern concept of Fitness* started to develop with Jogging and Jazzercise in the 1970s. The wireless heart rate monitor was invented by the founder of Polar in 1977. New companies came with digital computerized equipment mostly for the cardiorespiratory workout, making training sessions more user friendly. With Yoga and Pilates, one of today's concept of Wellness came in the 1990s, and functional training started to grow as a more integrated physical condition system among many other modern techniques, such as suspension training, core training, aqua-jogging, and so on. Even with the advancement of all these technologies, new sports, fitness products, informative and innovative devices to measure health, new training techniques in many health and fitness clubs, and so on, we were having a dominant sedentary lifestyle around the globe and a very low percentage of members in the clubs and gyms. According to the data from IHRSA in 2013, the average membership-retention rate was 66 percent, and I see too many clubs going out of business and too many getting into the market. However, the majority of people just don't work out; they do not even get physically active enough to have a healthier lifestyle.

This book, therefore, has brought you a solution for this problem.

Fourth Industrial Revolution (Industry 4.0, Since 2011)

Today, we live in this technological transformation that I had heard for the first time in 2015 from Klaus Schwab, the founder and executive chairman of the World Economic Forum (WEF). Cyber-physical systems, neurotechnological brain enhancements, the Internet of things, and the Internet of services, artificial intelligence, quantum computing, self-driving cars, and genetic editing are expanding importantly. The fusion of physical-digital and biological worlds is an important trend. The Smart World software is filling up our lives, showing perhaps a window that even though we, in general, are more physically inactive today, we could, with the help of all these new technologies directed to the right goal, make us more and more aware of the need to do more *Exercise*, giving us important data of our physical condition to track and process as never before, making visible in our hands and/or our eyes that which was invisible and unknown to us in the past, what with Biometrics coming fast, clear, and easy, helping us to change our bad and unhealthy habits. In 2014, the FIA Formula E Championship started in China (as a sustainable option for auto racing). In 2014, Alan Eustace set the record for the highest Free Fall Space Diving. By 2050, the Federation of International Robot-Soccer Association aims to create a team of robots capable of beating a human team in a football soccer match.

As these new technologies keep getting into the market, we are expecting a whole different sort of wearable products—4.0 Industry Health Monitors, Health Smart Apps, Training Machines, and so on—that have to face the global reality of a physically inactive, overweight, fat, and aging population in order to give them practical options to bring them into a more physically active and healthier way of living. In other words, this Industrial Revolution may be able to give us the solutions to the health problems that the previous Industrial Revolutions gave us as a side effect of modernity. But let's go beyond; let's see and bring the future. Of late, I have been listening to a German futurist, author and speaker, which my sister-in-law, Malena while she was working in EY (Ernst & Young), presented me through a video link that she sent me few weeks ago. His name is Gerd Leonhard, and he talks about very interesting subjects referring to the exponential change that technology as a tool is bringing to humanity. According to him, the Fourth Industrial Revolution is staggering. I want to write down now the mega-shifts that he thinks that the world is passing through today: digitization, mobilization, screenification, disintermediation, automation, intelligization, virtualization, anticipation, robotization. Why do I think these trends are important in the sports industry or, as I will call it, Wellness Industry? Because, I think, we can disrupt this industry applying them, for the benefit of all the stakeholders. Our body is an awesome asset, sustaining it well; enjoying all the experiences it can give us will make us more humans. A new type of intelligence is growing in our planet—artificial intelligence. This will compete with human intelligence more and more, to the point that it has been calculated that by the year 2048, it will be smarter than us (singularity point), and it is already competing with us today. Our biological body is something exclusive. To keep in the best condition that we can is a smart policy for everybody. To be alive is a miracle.

Let's enjoy it to the fullest!

CHAPTER 3

SPORTS MODEL TODAY

For me, losing a tennis match isn't failure; it's research.

—Billie Jean King

SPORTS MODEL TODAY

CHAPA WELLNESS MAP

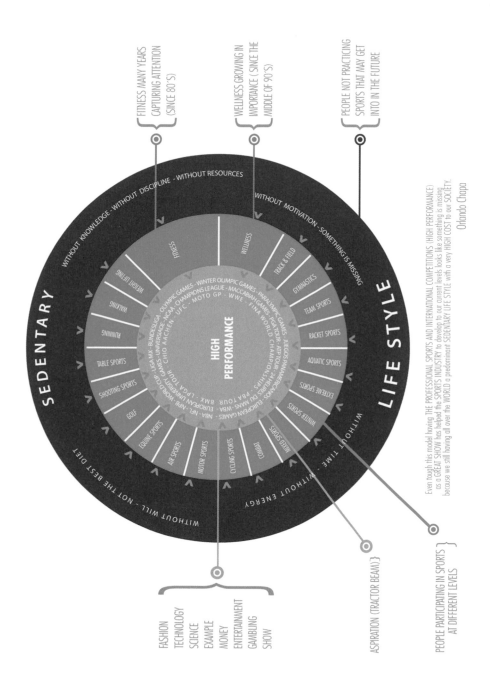

FITNESS MANY YEARS CAPTURING ATTENTION (SINCE 80'S)

WELLNESS GROWING IN IMPORTANCE (SINCE THE MIDDLE OF 90'S)

PEOPLE NOT PRACTICING SPORTS THAT MAY GET INTO IN THE FUTURE

WITHOUT KNOWLEDGE - WITHOUT DISCIPLINE - WITHOUT RESOURCES

WITHOUT MOTIVATION - SOMETHING IS MISSING

WITHOUT WILL - NOT THE BEST DIET

WITHOUT TIME - WITHOUT ENERGY

SEDENTARY

LIFE STYLE

HIGH PERFORMANCE

FITNESS
WELLNESS
TRACK & FIELD
GYMNASTICS
TEAM SPORTS
RACKET SPORTS
AQUATIC SPORTS
EXTREME SPORTS
WINTER SPORTS
MIXED SPORTS
COMBAT
CYCLING SPORTS
MOTOR SPORTS
AIR SPORTS
EQUINE SPORTS
GOLF
SHOOTING SPORTS
TABLE SPORTS
RUNNING
WALKING
WEIGHT LIFTING

OLIMPIC GAMES - WINTER OLIMPIC GAMES - PARALYMPIC GAMES - JUEGOS PANAMERICANOS - EUROPEAN GAMES - BUNDESLIGA - LIGA MX - WORLD CUP - NBA - NFL - NPB - MLB - WBA - ATP TOUR - WTA - 24 HEURES DU MANS - CHAMPIONS LEAGUE - MACCABIAH GAMES - FOR TOUR - PBA TOUR - BMX - LPGA TOUR - CHIO AACHEN - U.F.C. - MOTO GP - WWE - F.I.N.A WORLD CHAMPIONSHIPS - NCAA - UNIVERSIADE - EUROPEAN UNIVERSITY GAMES

Even tough this model having THE PROFESSIONAL SPORTS AND INTERNATIONAL COMPETITIONS (HIGH PERFORMANCE) as a GREAT SHOW has helped the SPORTS INDUSTRY to develop to our current levels looks like something is missing because we are still having all over the WORLD a predominant SEDENTARY LIFE STYLE with a very HIGH COST to our SOCIETY.
Orlando Chapa

FASHION
TECHNOLOGY
SCIENCE
EXAMPLE
MONEY
ENTERTAINMENT
GAMBLING
SHOW

ASPIRATION (TRACTOR BEAM) }

PEOPLE PARTICIPATING IN SPORTS AT DIFFERENT LEVELS

CONTEXT

This afternoon I jogged for one hour and walked for 30 minutes in a park that is 100 meters away from my apartment. I was running in the middle of trees, gardens, soccer, basketball, volleyball, and tennis courts. It reminded me of all the kids, girls, and adults who play some sport because they played it at school, or they are fans of the sport that they like, or they just want to feel good sweating and having fun with friends under the sun. This day also, I had to work deeper in this chapter, and again, I thought that is how sports have evolved until these days. But even though *Fitness* and *Wellness*, as they are understood today, keep growing in a positive direction, Physical Inactivity is the fourth cause of death globally, and I totally believe it is in our hands to make a disruptive change in order to bring an end to this problem, to cero (zero) deaths of physical inactivity soon. The model that I am presenting here—the *Chapa Wellness Map*—I really believe it can help to make this change in an important manner, and this chapter and the next are key to understand my concept. My hope is that all of you can grasp the idea of the model in a constructive and positive way, to use it for the good of all the inactive and active people all over the globe.

There is no doubt that the *Current Model of Sports* during all its development until today has brought to our society incredible good experiences, such as when our national soccer team wins a game in a world cup or with the design of new products as a skydiving parachute or with awesome athletes like Usain Bolt or with wireless technologies like polar monitors or with incredible stories like the mortal race of the messenger Philippides from Marathon to Athens in ancient Greece or with unforgettable flying legends as Michael Jordan or with pure talented professionals like Roger Federer or, in business, great companies like Adidas or with organizations like the Manchester United F.C. or with wise phrases like "When you win, say nothing. When you lose, say less" (Paul Brown) or with inspirational coaches like Vince Lombardy with the Green Bay Packers of the NFL or with attractive championships like the UEFA Champions League or with sport shows like Holiday on Ice or with top TV audience sports events as the Tour De France (2.6 billion audience) or with incredible architecture like the Allianz Arena stadium, with faithful fans to their professional team as those of the Argentinian Club Atlético Boca Juniors, or with millionaires like Many Pacquiao or with the promotion of fair play to encourage sportsmanship in international competitions, and so on.

On the other hand, the model has brought broken governments; for example, after organizing Olympic Games in 2004, Athens received almost 1 billion dollars from the Greek government, 97 percent over their planned budget, putting pressure to the economy of Greece; people who are in debt because of bad management gambling, betting in sports, represent 30 to 40 percent in the global gambling market; cheating professionals, who use steroids, like Lance Armstrong who was banned for life in 2012 from sanctioned Olympic sports and was voided of his seven Tour de France victories; corrupt sports leaders like in the FIFA (e.g., in 2015, FIFA President Sepp Blatter and UEFA President Michel Platini were banned for eight years from all football-related activities); dishonest coaches in universities paying to "amateur" student athletes, to the point that there exists a debate today about legalizing the payment to college athletes in the United States; and so on. But the bad thing that caught my attention the most is that, nevertheless, millions of dollars are invested and spent in the promotion of sports, professional sports and in their media, world sports events, sports products, sports facilities, and so on. Our lifestyle in society is mostly *Sedentary*, and the evident effects of this is the *Cost of Physical Inactivity* as presented in chapter 1 of this book. We have seen that industrial revolutions have played an important role in this situation, giving us less physically active lives in the workplace.

Therefore, my objective is to present the *Model of Sports as it is today*, in the way that I perceive it (after my involvement as a sports entrepreneur for 28 years, attending to more than 80 international sports trade shows worldwide since 1990; playing competitive international tennis (1985–1987); being a tennis coach (1986–1988); working as a fitness-equipment manufacturer (1987–1991); owning and managing a fitness center (1989–1990); working as a fitness-product manager (1991–1994); being a fitness-products developer and wholesaler to retail stores (1995–2018); being an importer and distributor of sports, fitness, and wellness products to health and fitness clubs (1987–1991 and 2002–2018); and studying marketing, economics, business strategy, hermeneutics, logic, apologetics, and so on, in different universities and colleges around the world).

The answer to the question as to where we are today will be given in chapter 3. After that, with the proposal of a new model, based on new definitions of the concepts of *Wellness* and *Fitness* and their relationship with the concept of *High Performance,* I will answer the following question in chapter 4: Where should we go?

I will try to answer these two questions within the context of the last paragraph and also consider two more questions: How do people get involved in sports today? What is the level of intensity or performance that people have at any moment while doing any physical activity or sport? To explore the answers basically, I see and present three main segments in our current sports model: High-Performance Athletes, Sports Active People, and Sedentary Lifestyle People (see graphic Sports Model Today).

HIGH-PERFORMANCE ATHLETES

When I was 15 years old, I started to play tennis when I saw the American John McEnroe defeat the Swedish Björn Borg in the tournament of Wimbledon in July 1981. What a great match! John took revenge from the previous year. I remember a famous Mexican TV commentator saying, "The King is dead, long live King!" Since that day, I started to go with a friend to the closest tennis court to play there or in the open spaces around my mother's apartment in Mexico City. But I was lucky, for the next month I had to go to my new school; I had been accepted to the agronomy high school in Chapingo, which is in the same campus of the university (UACH), which was around one and a half hours' drive from Mexico City back in 1981, where, fortunately for me, there was a tennis team and free tennis court for the students. I was excited, so I started to learn and play three times a week until my tennis coach (Sergio) told me I could go every day. I don't know how it all happened, but when I was 16 years old, I was becoming the number-one player of the high school, and I had started to play tournaments after just one year of my first tennis practice; it was then that I decided I wanted to be the number-one player of the world. I was a teenager with many dreams (maybe this was too going far, but for me it was so strong in my heart and mind on those days that it became the only thing that mattered in my life, so let's keep with the history).

The next year after that decision and after practicing tennis from two to four hours a day, I defeated a player who was three years older than me, who was the number one of the university; I was in my third and last high school year then. It was then that I decided to quit school, stop going to the university in Mexico, and go to live in the United States (San Antonio, Texas) to practice full-time tennis and to learn English. That period (1984–1985) was great, living for my dream by myself; maybe getting a scholarship in the short term could help, but, above all, I wanted to play professional tennis. I saw great college tennis matches there between San Antonio's Trinity University versus SMU, TCU, University of Texas at Austin, and so on. I was playing six hours a day at the McFarlin Tennis Center, doing my physical training, and I was feeling better and better with my game every day, so I decided to go back to Mexico to test how my game had improved by playing the national money tournaments, travelling and training with some friends around the country. It was difficult at first, as many good players were in the circuit, and sometimes we played the ATP satellite circuit and challenger tournament's qualifying rounds. It was tough for everybody; many good international players of the world ranked around the 150th. I remember the second round of the qualification in the ATP Challenger of San Luis Potosí, Mexico, in 1986; I played against the 200 ATP player of the world, Michael Fancutt from Australia. I was 19, and he was 25, and I gave one of the best games of my life; the score was a 6/4–6/4 victory for him. At the end of the match, he told me that was too hot and that my serve was jumping too high into his backhand, even though we were playing on clay, and that that was the reason why it was so hard for him to break my serve. It was just four and a half years since I played tennis as a beginner in Chapingo, and the demands technically, physically, and economically were high. My mom was alone, with only little help from my siblings, and not able to help me financially above basic needs like food, local transportation, balls, strings, tennis shoes, and so on, because my father had died when I was five years old; also, I had no coach, not too much budget to travel, and travelled and slept by night in the bus instead of flights to tournaments, hotels, and so on; but I was fighting my dream, trying to take on the world as a teenager. I was a low-level High-Performance Athlete.

One day in 1986, in a tournament in Manzanillo, a friend of mine who was a tennis player, having once beaten the 150 ATP–ranked player of the world, invited me to play the summer season of the French money tournaments in Toulouse. My family gave me the money, and I took another tennis player with me as a partner. We had booked the cheapest flight from New York to London, but prior to that I had to go from Mexico City to Atlanta by bus to practice for one week with another friend who had played college tennis in a good university in Georgia. I bought two Kneissl rackets there. I practiced for a week there. I had some fun with my friends and then left by bus to JFK Airport in New York; then by flight to London, Heathrow; then by train to Dover Port; and then ferried to Calais, France to take a train again to Paris, where we got our affiliation to the Fédération Francaise de Tennis, which is in the same facility where the Roland Garros Tournament is played. It was exciting to see the central stadium, to finally arrive at Toulouse. All that was about nine days of trip. Here, another friend, who was the touring pro of a tennis and rugby club in Toulouse, received us; another two Mexican tennis players were already there, and we started to practice and get rid of the jet lag, getting ready to fight in the tennis court almost for our lives. The budget was short, the competition was hard, and many South American Davis Cup players played here, looking to earn money to go to play satellite and challenger tournaments to gain ATP points and higher level so as to get into the ATP Grand Prix circuit of those days, the tournaments that are broadcasted in TV.

So we started to travel to the south of France by train—Carcassonne, Nimes, Montpellier, and so on. To my surprise, the level was tougher, even with the local French players. The competition system of France generates many good players, plus the ones from other countries. For us with a short budget, who had the dream and desire but had the need to win to earn some money, the results were almost catastrophic in the first tournaments, even though I had beaten my friend once in practice, the one with some important victories over ATP-ranked players around the 150. So the weeks kept going, and I don't remember how, but at some point we had separated (my Mexican partners and I), and soon I was travelling first with a new friend from South Africa, who was a varsity player at

THE **CHAPA WELLNESS MAP**

LSU (Louisiana State University) and was top ranked in his country when he was a junior. A few weeks later, I was travelling with another new friend from Brazil, who was in the top 15 professionals of his country. Here, another High-Performance adventure happened to meet me; after losing both in another French tournament, he told me, "Let's go to Austria to play an ATP Grand Prix qualifying," so we took the train to Kitzbühel. It was a long ride but was interesting passing through France and Switzerland. Finally, we arrived in Austria, to this beautiful town; to my surprise, the tournament was the 12th most important tournament of the highest circuit of tennis in the world and was the Austrian Open on clay. So we got accepted to play, and soon I was there in the players' lounge having some fresh water with Guillermo Vilas, Miroslav Mecir, Joakim Nystrom, Andres Gomez, and other top world players. But I was just a player of the qualifying rounds and surely one of the weakest. Also, I found another friend, the number-three professional player of Mexico, Hector Ortiz (RIP); he was in a much higher level as a tennis player than me, but he invited me to practice. He was nice; he was always a very kind person. So after much excitement around, I had to play my match, and, you know, it was very hard, as the clay was heavy. I had a good serve and used to go to the net all the time. I played against an Austrian specialist on clay, but as I was not good from the baseline, he defeated me easily. I was 20 years old then, and all the odds were against me as a professional tennis player, but it was worth it. I came back to Mexico in the middle of another adventure. Money was always short, but I made it back home safe. During the next year, 1986–1987, I had financial pressure in family and pressure to go back to school because I had an injured knee and had always been a good student; so I started to teach tennis and help my family at the gym that they owned and then I got back to the university, now taking up economics, with an academic scholarship at the Mexican private university, ITAM. I was virtually retired as High-Performance tennis player in June 1987, at the age of 21. Therefore, *to me, as Billie Jean has said, losing is research, so here I am.*

My professional tennis career was really a failure in terms of winning matches, tournaments, and money; but, you know, it helped me to have a risk-taking character that was good for business and many other skills. I learned English, and some French as well, but I also got a bit of the taste of the world of High-Performance Sports. Can you imagine all the stories? Not just of the great champions that we know but also of those millions of people like me all over the globe, in so many sports, who have had all kinds of experiences of victories and failures, shattered dreams due to injuries, triumph by persistence, and tears of emotion and despair. Every mind is a world. Today's Sports Model is great in many fields; I can testify of that with my heart and soul, but as we have started to analyze in this book, we need to be improve it and maybe in a disruptive way.

Now, getting back to definitions, we can say that in this category, we have the professionals and amateurs of the higher level of physical condition. To be attractive as a show and as an aspiration for prospective clients, *"to be like the champion"* to buy equipment with the technology and specifications *"that the champion uses,"* may be the engine of our current model, as I see it, to motivate inactive people to practice sports and/or to consume sporting goods (in 2017 Nike's sales were of $34.35 billion dollars worldwide) and/or to be a spectator ($3.9 billion people tune in at some point the FIFA World Cup of 2014) as an example. This system, even though being incredibly successful in many ways, *has fallen short in activating people physically* all over the world.

One study that would be very useful to do in the short term is to answer the question, how does frustration affect kids' and teenagers' involvement in future physical activity when they find out that they cannot perform as their idols?. I believe that here we may find an important factor that perhaps brings some discouragement to many kids, teenagers, and maybe some adults who are not skilled enough for the sport they like to practice, because they cannot play as the High-Performance player that they try to follow and also that they just cannot play it at all. Such people tend to end their not-too-successful short "sports career" by drinking some beer and having pizza at any sports bar with some friends and feeling that to watch it is fun but to practice it is just too hard for them. I am not saying that this model is bad at all; we all know many motivating and encouraging stories of people of all ages who have overcome all kinds of obstacles to become champions, and this has inspired a good many people all over the world. However, I am searching where the *flaws* of the current model may be; this is not to criticize it in a destructive way but to look for options to improve it in a practical way, looking to the future, keeping the good and improving the things that are not working at their best.

PEOPLE ACTIVE IN SPORTS

Just by moving, the heart pumps more blood and increases the blood circulation in our bodies, more oxygen goes into our lungs, energy expenditure increases, fat and protein turn into glucose, brain cells function at higher levels, and endorphins are generated. Apart from these, more happens when we exercise just any given day of our lives. But if we keep moving for longer periods of time, we will have stronger and bigger muscles; the metabolism will increase as we burn more calories even during periods of rest; our capacity for more physical activity will increase; the brain will release more endorphins, and we will be feeling much better; and the activities of our daily life will become much easier. This is what physically active people enjoy. Also, since they keep doing it for weeks and months, they have their weight under control; their bodies generate more good cholesterol (HDL) and decreased unhealthy triglycerides; more brain chemicals help them feel happier and relaxed; they have better sleep; and they have more energy for family, work, study, love, social life, and so on. In general, they enjoy life in a complete manner.

These are the persons who are involved in one or more of many sports that are available today, and they are involved because it is fun for them, for their health, for relieving stress, socializing, doing business, competing, enjoying family time, and so on. Very few people, before the age of 12, because they may be very skilled in one or more sports and have the support of parents or/and coaches or/and government, may get involved in a more intensive program, looking to play that sport at High-Performance level at some time in the future, where some will make it and some not. On the other hand, some kids, teenagers, or adults just do not keep playing sports for many reasons, such as studies, work, sickness, injury, economy, sentiments, and so on, thereby reducing their physical activity, backsliding into a Sedentary Lifestyle; this is a pattern that generates health problems.

I want to highlight again two important concepts that, according to me, are not very well defined because they are not too old and change over time. In chapter 4, we will redefine them in the context of the *New Model* that we are presenting, which is *"Chapa Wellness Map."* These new conceptual definitions are the basis of this *"Systematic Approach to Physical Activity"* that I am explaining all over this book. These two concepts are *Fitness* and *Wellness*.

Fitness is defined today in the dictionary as "the state of being fit" (biology). In our Sports Model Today, it could also be defined as the Physical Activity that clusters together many other activities such as the step; spinning; weight training; jogging; running; boxing; suspension training; Zumba; core training; balance training; stability ball training; functional training; circuit training; aqua-jogging; and the use of free weights, integrated weight machines, treadmills, bicycles, rowers, steppers, elliptical trainers, Arc machines, and so on; and many more physical activities, also keeping a healthy and planned diet, taking protein supplements, amino acids, fat burners, energy busters, weight gain powders, and so on. All these are done to feel better, perform better, and have a good-looking body shape and a healthy physical and mental condition.

Some athletes perceive Fitness as the athletic preparation to be *"Fit"* for high-level competitions. Fitness started to grow as a concept with the nuance that is mostly related to the GYMs in the 1980s when videos came—like the Jane Fonda movies; many products in infomercials; the opening of many gyms like Gold's Gym; people running in races all over the cities; new concepts of treadmills in stores; models in TV and magazines as a living proof of the concept of being Fit; soccer, basketball, and tennis players looking more Fit on media; and more people socializing in fitness centers—to the point that talking of workouts keeping a healthy diet, not smoking, and not drinking was ok in the office, home, and friends.

Let's take a look at some business statistics. In 2017, the global fitness market has been calculated to be $82.1 billion dollars, with 187,000 health and fitness clubs worldwide having more than 151 million members and having LA Fitness as the top of the world chain in revenue with $1.912 billion. Very interesting industry, but I believe that it has to evolve.

The Wellness concept, as is in this *Sports Model Today*, started to sound strong in the market of the health and fitness industry in the mid-1990s, mostly with two old but fast-growing techniques such as yoga and Pilates, including massage, SPAs, organic and bio food, vegan lifestyle, meditation, baby workouts, senior training systems, and so on. So, as I perceive, the use of the concept of Wellness today refers basically to a group of activities and good habits that look basically for good health, antiaging, life-span extension, relaxation, and stress relief, among many other benefits, for a better way of living. Also, it sounds clear that Wellness, the condition of being well, incorporates everything that helps you to be in a good or better condition physically and mentally. Very interesting and evolving industry.

In the past few years, I have seen that health clubs are relating this concept more and more to health programs like weight reduction as in the YMCAs of the United States. In 2016, I met a friend in Slovenia, who is the director of Cardiac Rehabilitation and Wellness Cardiology in Mayo Clinic in Scottsdale, Arizona. The company, Technogym, in Italy, is a leading manufacturer of machines and accessories for commercial use, and the home market has as its corporative statement "the wellness company," and they are doing a great job, creating state-of-the-art machines and accessories. However, we also see the concept assigned to almost every SPA in every nice hotel in the world, and for many it means a body-mind connection in activities like yoga, Pilates, and mindfulness. We also see kids and seniors around the concept of Wellness in magazines and advertisings and billboards in health clubs. So the concept, as I see it, has been changing and maturing but not defined well yet.

If we check some Wellness Industry statistics, we can find that it has a current value of 3.7 trillion dollar market. What? We found that Fitness claims a market of $80.2 billion; this is because we have here the sauna market, beauty, some art, spas architecture, comfortable cancer-recovering programs, and so on. I agree all that gives us Well-Being and Wellness, and this is the logic of the market and the industry and has worked pretty well so far. But we are having a huge problem: 6 percent of global yearly deaths is due to Physical Inactivity. This is the reason I wrote the book, to try to understand better these concepts so as to help find a solution for this situation, and, you know, I think we can find it! I see in the future many people in the world living longer and better because of the fruits of this and many others working. We will get back to these *key concepts—Wellness, Fitness, and High Performance*—in the next chapter of this book, where I will redefine them for the New Model.

SEDENTARY LIFESTYLE PEOPLE

Let's say that we sleep daily for eight hours, spend about half an hour for showering and dressing, work eight hours, and spend about one and a half hours for going to and coming back from the office, two hours for eating, one hour for family time, and one and a half hours for reading and personal time. Now we have just one and a half hours left for many options around. Where do we find the time to go to the gym or to the park to run? This is one of the reasons why I think it is too hard to get involved in Physical Activity. If we want to leave the *Sedentary Lifestyle* to have a better and longer life, we must be good managers of our time and give priority to physical activity, because our body needs it, but our culture seems not to. This is starting to change; it is obvious, as we see more and more advertisings pro-corporal activity but requires too much social energy to make the shift to a *Physically Active Culture*. This is worthy, and the main winners of this possible change are us.

To have an idea of our cultural situation today, we have around 80 percent of worldwide kids inactive; but on the other hand, the number-one product we have in sales is the PlayStation by Sony with 344 million units sold since it was introduced into the market since 1995 (data of 2014). This is a great product that has given entertainment and happy moments to many in the family and with friends, but it is a clear example of where the interest of kids is. The product that has been sold the most in those 19 years is not a ball of soccer or basketball where you have to move to use it; we need video games oriented to make the children and adults move. Last April at FIBO 2018 in Cologne, Germany, I saw two companies from Finland presenting Pro-Activity Video Games for the commercial market, and they are innovative, of high quality, and effective but a little expensive, because they are made for the clubs, schools, malls, and so on, not for home use. The second product with more sales in history is Lipitor, by Pfizer, with $141 billion dollars since its introduction to the market in 1997. What does Lipitor do? It lowers the levels of LDL or bad cholesterol. I think it is great that the research in the laboratories has brought this pharmaceutical product to help people to reduce the risk of heart diseases, but it also makes us realize how inadequate our Physical Activity is and how bad our diet is, because most of the people who exercise regularly and eat healthy food have good cholesterol levels. We have many other diseases that affect us and will affect us as we grow older, so if we can reduce the expenses in physical inactivity/bad-diet-related diseases, the pharmaceutical companies could focus on new drugs for those diseases without losing revenue, and we could save budget to meet other health demands that for sure we will face. In this manner, we will be building a smarter market for everybody, don't you agree?

In this category, we find people who do not practice any sport or indulge in Physical Activity, beyond the one that the normal daily living activity brings, and as we have seen, it has been decreasing with modern times. For many reasons, some people practice some sport or Physical Activity, but soon they stop doing it; yet, in some parts of the world, people may not practice any sport at all. In western culture, perhaps due to the lack of time, too much time behind an electronic screen, too much time sitting at work, or passive socialization, and so on, there are many bad effects on the health of the people. Again, I am not saying that any of these conditions are bad in their core; I am trying to say that too much time doing that may bring them health problems. This lifestyle—*Sedentarism*—contributes to many preventable causes of death, as we have seen in the Cost of Physical Inactivity revised in Chapter 1. As I pointed out at the beginning of this chapter, the size of this population segment worldwide is perhaps the most harmful effect of our *Sports Model Today*; we have more than 30 percent of adults and 80 percent of kids not doing enough sports or physical activity. It is something that has to open our eyes and mind to make a change.

Something has to be done!

CHAPTER 4

CHAPA WELLNESS MAP: BE ACTIVE, BE WELL, BE ALIVE

Sports promotion must converge to Wellness and diverge to High-Performance.

—Orlando Chapa

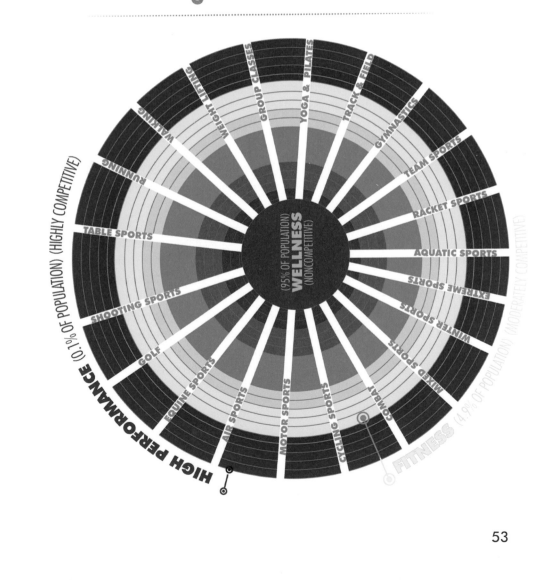

CHAPA WELLNESS MAP

A MODEL FOR SPORTS SUSTAINABILITY

"Sports promotion must converge to WELLNESS and diverge to HIGH PERFORMANCE"

Orlando Chapa

STORY OF DEVELOPMENT

In 1987, when I started to manufacture fitness equipment in my own club (Zovek High Tech Gym, 1989–1990) and in my family's fitness center (Zovek Club & Gym, 1984–1991), I realized that something was very different there compared to the sports that I liked and practiced the most—American football (where I played as quarterback three seasons in two teams) and tennis (where I gave my life to it for six years and the last three for more than six hours a day). Maybe since I was a baby then (1966), I was used as a dumbbell for my father's workout (Francisco Javier Chapa Del Bosque "Zovek"). Something was different around these activities that I found in the trendy opening of gyms everywhere; something was special. I wondered why?. Almost all friends of mine who were football players and, of course, the professionals and college players, including tennis players, needed to work out in the gym to be more competitive in their sport, and this was not the same way inversely; I mean, not too many people working out in the Fitness Centers played American football or tennis to be better or more competitive. Therefore, I started to wonder whether something special was going on there. I said to myself, "Fitness is not a common group of activities. Fitness is in some way more structural than any other sport or group of sports." With this, I wanted to say that it was more fundamental or essential, looking to sports as a whole.

In 1990, I traveled to my first international sporting goods trade show—the Super Show—in Atlanta, Georgia. I was manufacturing gym equipment and managing my own gym in Mexico City, now CDMX, so I decided to look for opportunities to export equipment there. I was 23 years old then, so that experience was incredible for me. More than 80,000 visitors had come, in 1991; the expected attendance was 88,000, to the most important trade show of sporting goods in the world back in those days. I saw stands of many brands—Adidas, Nike, Reebok, Wilson, K-Swiss, New Balance, LA Gear, Lifefitness, Cybex, Paramount, Universal, Marcy, Soloflex, Prince, Babolat, Head, License Products (NFL, NBA, NHL, MBL, NCAA), Polar, Vectra, Weider, Proform, and many, many, many more. I was impacted with all the marketing used in the stands to present the new products and with the design and technology of the majority of the new products; but, above all, *I saw for the first time in my life in just one shot the complete Sports Industry, the big picture!*

Coming back, I found the reality of the Mexican market; not too many of those imported products were sold, and I was having good orders of professional gym equipment made in Mexico by my small company. My gym was not doing very well; it was small, and I did not have all the investment required to give the best service. It was good as a showroom to sell equipment, but in my head, many ideas of how to improve my equipment popped up after that trip. So without knowing, I was specializing everyday more and more in the Fitness Industry. That year I had to close my Fitness Center because the rent was increased the double, but I kept as a manufacturer and moved with my brother Francisco to his gym, that was five blocks away from mine. There I had my new showroom and office for one year. In those days I was in love and that relationship required a good financial support from me, that I did not have because I was always giving me a low salary to have more profits reinvest, so I had too much pressure between business and love, and finally, after not having the opportunity to buy the license for Mexico of the most important fitness brand in Mexico, I decided to work for a company, looking for stability, because of my loving relationship. Uff!

So, in 1991, I was hired as the Fitness Divisional Manager of the Mexican leading sporting goods stores chain named Deportes Martí, which required also to be the product manager of the York Barbell Brand in Mexico. I always had in my head the idea that Fitness must go in one way or the other in the center of the industry for many technical, conceptual, commercial, and practical reasons, and today I can say for *Systematic reasons,* too. Those years were awesome, three to be precise, until the year of 1994; there I also got involved in the initial stages with the project that was going to be the most important chain of health and fitness clubs in Mexico for more than 20 years, Sport City. I just want to say thank you to all the people who allowed me to be part of those projects, which was very important in my life; thank you from the depth of my heart and for respect to that company. This is all that I am going to write about that period of my life in this book.

The University California, Berkeley, gave me great vision in strategic management, back in 1994, when I took a six-month executive program with excellent teachers. There I learned about strategic tools to do analysis, like the BCG Matrix (Boston Consulting Group Matrix), where I understood about what we can get with the combination of two variables, in this case Relative Market Share versus Industry Growth, where we can clearly see why a product is a Star, such as an iPhone, or as the GE Matrix (General Electric Matrix) that is similar to using Industry Attractiveness instead of Industry Growth, where we can see if it is convenient to Invest or to Retire. These tools also inspired me many years later to develop *the Chapa Wellness Map that I can define as a strategic tool for the sports industry.* It was a good program at Berkeley.

In 1995, being vegetarian, practicing yoga and going all over Mexico to mystical places to do all kinds of meditations, I was founding with my sister Holistic Fitness, trying to find new and creative ways to develop new products through the fusion of Body, Mind, and Spirit. Here I saw a new English concept coming into the market in those days—Wellness—many times related to yoga, Pilates, sauna, kids, seniors, nature, and so on. Since that time, I had always perceived Wellness in some way as a lighter Fitness, more for seniors, kids, and not to a too-high-intensity workout people. The concept of Wellness itself lodged in my mind with a strong impression.

In 1996, Mexico was just about to recover from a severe national economic crisis that started in December 1994, noticing the need to develop the Health Conservancy markets and watching the saturation of many Fitness Products (home treadmills, elliptical machines, bikes, steppers, empty infomercials, etc.) looking for a different distribution channel, through drug stores. It was then that I created the ES 3 BALL brand (Stress Ball, three sounds TRES in Spanish), with the aim of helping people in preventing the growing number of incidences of carpal tunnel syndrome, a degenerative disease of the hand caused in many cases by excessive use of keyboards, and, as its name says, helping people to do some exercise with the hand as a way to handle stress. So I was building my first Wellness brand and a clear example of an exerciser of today's worldwide movement, Exercise is Medicine.

From 1997 to 2002, my best client of Fitness Equipment was Sears Roebuck Mexico. I remember that I saw an opportunity in the market to help Sears to compete against other specialist companies in Fitness. I made a proposal to develop for them a private label highlighting the competitive advantage of Sears versus the sport specialists, and that was the *home;* yes, Sears had everything for the home that the sport specialist stores didn't. So making a brand bringing the gym to home in a more lighter, warm, and cozy way, I could now say with my model in a more *Wellness Way*, because the competitors were more sportive, harder, and tougher. But do you know what happened? I never got the chance to present it to the higher levels of management, so that idea was just kept in PowerPoint in my 1998 Hewlett Packard computer.

In 2002, I was living in Cuernavaca, a city full of tennis courts. The economy was a little bit slow in Mexico City, and even though I had had good sales of treadmills and other Fitness products to Walmart and Sears Roebuck Mexico the years before, I had to move to Cuernavaca because sales were slow for me again. There finally I had the opportunity to implement an Innovative Tennis Class—"*Diet Tennis*"—an idea that had been in my head since 1990, because of the huge media presence of the Diet and Light colas back in those years. I said to myself, "Yes! I could make a sport more attractive with a different marketing approach combining Tennis and Fitness." I taught with a friend a small group of women for about a month; let's say that was my laboratory, and it was very good, but you know me—that was just another experience to keep going for a bigger project. So there I was, already applying a model that had been growing inside my head for many years but was not so clear to me yet. So, without knowing and just by watching, analyzing, and getting new personal skills with time, experiences, and studies, the solution was going to come to me someday by drawing it on a paper—the solution for a model that could make

Fitness but was not Fitness, now I can say, the center and the core of all sports industry looking to integrate or activate all the people of the world, to make in some way, the Theory of Everything for sports.

In 2007, I was developing the Zovek Balance Ball, a gym ball under my father's image (see Zovek in glossary). I realized that I needed three main segments—in other words, three different levels of thickness in the balls: Home, Club and Gym, and High- Performance. To be clear, a gym ball made with a not-too-heavy material for light use at home (lower cost); a gym ball with the resistance of material for heavy-duty use at gyms and clubs (medium cost); and a gym ball for the Xtreme user, very heavy material for the athlete (higher cost). I got insights to solve questions that I was asked myself back in 1987. The launching of this product was never done because the doors were not open with my key target clients, but I was learning new things.

From 2007 to 2012, I got deep into theological studies, leaving my business in the freezer half of the time, three months of study in Germany and three months of work in my business in Mexico. I was reading many books and attending classes to learn hermeneutics, logic, apologetics, ancient Greek, systematic theology, homiletics, among many other subjects. My mind was getting sharp handling very fine concepts, reading about the way of thinking of very interesting disruptive authors (Saint Augustine, Martin Luther, John Calvin, Jonathan Edwards), doing research to write papers and to present them speaking to the public; visiting Jerusalem, Galilee, The Dead See, Patmos, Philippi, Corinth, Athens, Wittenberg, Worms, and Eisenach, doing my personal spiritual research. It was great! I was getting new skills that definitively helped me to finally grasp the model that had been running in my head for many years.

In 2012, back in Mexico after those five years studying and living half of the time mostly in Germany, answers to my questions as a model came to me clear: *three concentric circles having a Green Circle in the center with a new definition of the concept of Wellness; then a Yellow Circle in the Middle with a new definition of the concept of Fitness; and the final and most External Circle, color Red, with a new definition of the concept of High-Performance.* The reason why I draw it on a paper that way is, thinking that for almost everybody, the High-Performance level is a level of a very high intensity of any sport or a level of very high physical condition of people—in this particular case, the Highest, where the athletes are, who train hard for more than 20 hours a week and with the highest level of knowledge of applied sports science in their programs and with the highest resources of all kind in most of the countries worldwide. Then I started to think why not put ourselves at the same level in the model, at the structural level, at the level of intensity that any sport is performed, or at the level of the physical condition of any person? The next two concepts have had my attention almost 35 years (35 years for Fitness and 17 years for

Wellness as it was in 2012). If Wellness is a lighter Fitness, then Wellness would come in the center on Green, as in a traffic light. Why Green? Because we have to have a green light here to signal as a Go light for all the sectors that may have interest in this industry so that they may go there, invest there, and converge there. Why? Because it is not in the High-Performance level, the most Extreme Level, the Red One, where most of the people of the nations are, because it is not in the Middle Circle, the Fitness Circle (the Yellow Circle as I draw it) between Wellness and High-Performance, where all the well-shaped bodies are (Fit Bodies), where we do not have much of the population. It is in the Central Circle (as I designed it), the Origin Circle, where we all start at some point in our lives, where our level of intensity of physical activity, where we practice any sport, (in case that we do practice one), is minimal and from here starts to grow to a better Wellness Zone if we start to move more. This is where our physical condition has to be improved as soon as possible so as to reduce the risk of many diseases and deaths. *Here is where the majority of the world population are—the Sedentary Level—and has to start to move up to improve in the classification level.* Thus, *we must go Green, we must be Well, we must go Wellness,* as I have presented in this book.

In retrospect, when I decided to write this book to present the model, I did notice that the Chapa Wellness Map Concentric Circles Model was the antithesis of the Current Sports Model in the way that I had perceived the Sports Industry until that time. So I needed to make map it out to write the book; I needed to make the Thesis (chapter 3) to better explain the Antithesis (chapter 4), knowing that the next chapters of the book were going to be the Synthesis using the Hegelian Triad to explain part of my methodology.

So on May 8, 2013, I decided to place the first concentric circles model design on my business "Bienestar Sustentable" (Sustainable Wellness) webpage to share this idea with more people, but something was missing. People were not clearly understanding the concept, so I started to develop more maps (chapters 5 and 6), and it was then I realized that I needed to write a book.

During 2013 and 2014, the chain of clubs Sport City in Mexico, started to buy me many products for group classes, physical conditioning, and other such stuff. I was very busy attending them until the Mexican peso started to depreciate with respect to the dollar up to almost 50 percent. So in 2015, my business went down drastically, and I started to write this book, travelling to Germany, Switzerland, Spain, Slovenia, Italy, and the United States and visiting universities, trade shows, symposiums, family, friends, and my publisher in Aachen, Germany. Finally I wrote the book in Germany and Mexico between 2015 and 2018; in those years, I declined many projects that had distracted me a bit before, and I am closing my business now as I am writing these lines, to dedicate myself full time to the book, to promote its concepts and ideas, making things happen, to write more books, and to look which doors are open to accomplish the goals established in this *Be Active, Be Well, Be Alive* book.

We will see during the development of the coming paragraphs and chapters that this central Wellness Circle is not just the sedentary level but goes to a level where our health could be in a very safe place. Even though we may not get to the Fitness level, we may get to a very interesting level that I will define better in chapter 9.

Now, I am going to define these three concepts under this New Map so that we may get better understanding of them and, most important, how we can apply this Systematic Approach on the development of the industry and, as our *Top Priority, how we can increase the levels of Wellness by Physical Activity of the people worldwide*—in other words, how we can give to each person in the world a better and longer life.

Be Active, Be Well, Be Alive.

WELLNESS (W)

As I have defined in the Chapa Wellness Map, a person's wellness level is the level and performance of physical activity or the level of physical conditioning from the lowest possible (as an office worker who sits almost all day long, who drives to get to work, who on weekends doesn't do any sport or physical activity, who doesn't pay any attention to diet, etc.) up to a point just under a person's current fitness level. At this point in the Wellness model, a person has reduced all the risks of contracting any disease related to Physical Inactivity. He can be confident that because of having done the recommended Physical Activity and because of a healthy diet, the odds of getting heart disease, type 2 diabetes, colon and breast cancer, among other diseases have been minimized considerably; we can say that the statistics are on their side. The main values of Wellness that I present and that we will see deeper in chapter 5 are feeling good, having good health, relaxation, stress release, weight loss, life-span extension, having fun, socializing, learning, less time required for doing physical activity, among others. Here is where most of the world population is, and in this model, I have divided in 10 segments, they being the initial W1 and the final W10 (see map in chapter 8). Here I have defined a special segment from W7 to W10, "The Wellness Sweet Spot," where the person who has reached this point in his Physical Condition Level has reduced his risk to get diseases related to Physical Inactivity in the healthiest way. I am sure that this level is easier to get and to sustain for the majority of the world's population compared to a higher level, the Fitness Level, which requires more economical resources and personal efforts that are not and will not be available in the coming future for most of the population of the world. This is the reason why I have labeled this model as a Model for Sports Sustainability. Also, we have here the great advantage that at this level, it is harder to get injured or to be burned out because of overtraining. The Sporting Goods, Fitness and Wellness companies, just have to keep the fun and a high attractiveness within the activities and products offered to this market segment so that people can keep moving up in the Wellness Map for better levels of physical condition—in other words, for a better and longer life.

So we have a more reachable state, Wellness redefined. In order to become more physically active, we have to enrich our physical activities with creativity, innovation, research, pragmatism, and more promotion and *make Wellness more Tangible*, because it is not as it is in Fitness (where you can see a body totally changed from the outside and people can see it). Many of the benefits of this level are not easy to see and are in some way hidden as blood chemistry correct numbers (cholesterol, triglycerides), aerobic condition, body mass index, body-fat percentage, waist circumference, waist-hip ratio, and so on; but are evident for the person who has increased his levels of Wellness by Physical Activity, because that person feels better physically and mentally.

FITNESS (F)

Here I am redefining the concept of *Fitness* for this model, and it is where people have the condition of being Fit, completely Fit, Totally Fit, because they have the right body-fat percentage, correct body mass index, right waist circumference, correct waist-hip ratio, correct aerobic condition, blood chemistry correct numbers (cholesterol, triglycerides) that are required in the Wellness Levels, and good body symmetry, good levels of strength, endurance, speed, balance, coordination, flexibility, and power that are in the Fitness Levels. I am presenting five levels of Fitness, from F1 to F5 (see graph in chapter 8). Here we have the people who, through working-out sessions, right nutrition, discipline, time, knowledge, effort, sweat, money, methodology, and so on, have gotten a body that looks good (with other people noticing it) and have enough knowledge of their body, training techniques, diet, exercise equipment, and so on, that many of them become instructors to others. The main qualitative values of Fitness that I am defining (see map in chapter 5) are image, shape, discipline, advice, teaching, challenging, profession, perfection, part-time, among others.

I have placed Fitness in this model between the Wellness and High-Performance levels. One of the main differences compared with the people at Wellness level is that here in Fitness level, the people have a symmetrical Shape, they look good, and they have a good image. The main difference with the people at High-Performance level is that at this level, they are amateurs or professionals, who represent, through competition, either themselves or their countries, teams, schools, universities, clubs, and so forth.

Compared to Wellness, Fitness is harder to attain and harder to sustain for everybody; it is good for people who are self-driven into sports or are physically active but not so good for the others. From an economical, national, and global perspective too, it is not the best because of the resources required. It is a good aspiration but not feasible to attain for everybody. Therefore, many may get frustrated at some point, because media sells Fitness, but few can reach it, so the majority of people may feel better by not getting involved in sports or physical activity, because they perceive and have experienced that they were not made for that, so they may conclude that the only relationship with sports they may get in the future is as spectators, thereby backsliding into a Sedentary Lifestyle, just as it has happened with the sports model of the great champion that many were not able to become, which we analyzed in chapter 3. So we have here two important concepts that have given, and still give, great benefits to many, but that can't retain everybody in physical activity and sports, Fitness and High-Performance. This point is key on the Chapa Wellness Map Model.

HIGH-PERFORMANCE (HP)

This is the highest-level physical activity or physical condition that is attained after many years of intensive physical training and strict exercise accompanied by a strict diet, among many other high-level resources. To grasp this zone better, I present the qualitative values (see map in chapter 5) of this level; they are invention, idol, icon, example, champion, records, professionalism, representation, full time, among others. I have placed it in the External Circle in Red Color because I believe that we have promoted sports too much from the High-Performance level (see map in chapter 7), displaying the Sport Rock Star all over the media so that people may want to be like him and, as I have commented before, has been good but not good enough because of the bad numbers that we have, as we have seen in the Cost of Physical Inactivity (Chapter 1). And we haven't displayed the Wellness Level enough in media, as we are understanding this concept only now.

I am assigning five circles, five sections for this level, from High-Performance 1 (HP 1), where we may have here a high-school or a university athlete who represents his team, up to High-Performance 5 (HP 5), where I have placed the Top of the Top, the best sports professionals and athletes of all times, such as Michael Jordan, Roger Federer, Greg Louganis, Lionel Messi, Zovek, and so on (see map in chapter 8).

The time required every week for a person with the right skills is 20 hours or more of intensive and high-intensive training to get and stay at High-Performance level. For Fitness level, a person with the correct skills may need to invest between 10 and 20 hours of weekly physical activity/sports. To be at the Wellness level, a person doing physical activity or not doing it may need between ZERO and 10 hours a week. Let's remember that the Goal at Wellness and the minimal aspiration for any person who wants to have more possibilities to keep healthy and live better is *The Wellness Sweet Spot* (see map in chapter 9) and that the amount of hours invested in doing physical activity is not the only factor required to achieve one level or another; this factor could only give us an initial idea (see map in chapter 8).

SOME APPLICATIONS

Another application of the Chapa Wellness Map is that we can very clearly see the three main levels of Physical Condition as a base for a New Sports Industry Model, and above this base we can put all the sports. I have placed 19 divisions that hold more than 300 sports that any of them could be played at Wellness, Fitness, or High-Performance. This model could help product designers, inventors, product managers, marketing managers, personal trainers, entrepreneurs, and so on, to develop all kinds of products and services with this particular approach. As an example, I have developed using this map Wellness Tennis, Yoga-Walk, and Wellness Kid Toy, which I am planning to launch into the market in the future.

Now, let's suppose that the product manager of a tennis brand wants to develop a tennis racket with a disruptive approach, to promote physical activity among kids through tennis all over the world. Let's say that Roger Federer agrees to endorse it because we have 80 percent of the kids physically inactive, and we know that he loves to support these types of causes, so the manager decides to build up a Wellness Racket, according to the strategic management tool Chapa Wellness Map, to develop a specific motor skill on the kids while helping them to move more, have fun, and learn tennis. Let's say that Roger Federer wants to improve the kids' reaction, so the product manager asks the production manager for a prototype racket with some liquid gel inside the racket frame that adds some moving weight to the racket, which is neither too heavy nor full of it such that the liquid flows all over the racket while the kid tries to hit the ball. Thus, *this racket seems to be Alive*; it has trick, and the kid needs to put more attention to control it, compared to other rackets. The kid has fun, while being more active and learning how to play a sport. With this racket, the kid could simulate his or her tennis strokes without the ball and without a tennis court that in many countries may not be easy to have. Just by fighting a bit with this crazy Wellness Racket, the kid will be increasing his physical activity and developing his ability to react. Roger Federer will be very happy seeing more kids being active, skilled, and less obese all around the world, playing the sport that he loves. The product manager gets a promotion, and the tennis brand will keep his leadership with innovation that matters. Of course, this is a total conceptual invention that I just thought and wrote, just to give you an example of how the Chapa Wellness Map could be used in business—in this particular case to develop a product. Soon I will write another book with 100 new business innovative ideas so that we can help to achieve the goals established in this first book.

Another application that we will see in a practical and more detailed way in Special Topics of this book is to locate our position in the Chapa Wellness Map—in other words, what is our level of physical condition in a practical and clear manner, to know where we are, and to know where we should go, according to our objectives or at least to be in a position where the risks of getting a disease related with physical inactivity has been reduced. The key point for anybody here is to get out as soon as possible from the first three lower levels—W1, W2, and W3—that are the Sedentary Lifestyle Levels (see map in chapter 8), meaning our physical activity is below the recommended one by the World Health Organization or below the recommended one by our physician. We need to get out quickly from this area of the Chapa Wellness Map, because here is where the health problems may take us by surprise. You can get your preliminary level on the Special Topics section at the end of this book, namely, "Do you want to know your Wellness Level? Get it now, or contact us at orlando@chapawellnessmap.info." Soon I will write a book that will be totally focused on how you can practically know your level and improve it in this classification system at the workplace.

CHAPTER 5

CHAPA WELLNESS MAP: QUALITATIVE VALUES

The real voyage of discovery consists not in seeking new landscapes, but seeing with new eyes.

—Marcel Proust

CHAPA WELLNESS MAP
QUALITATIVE VALUES

WELLNESS | YOU FEEL GOOD

FITNESS | YOU LOOK GOOD

HIGH PERFORMANCE | YOU REPRESENT GOOD

Orlando Chapa

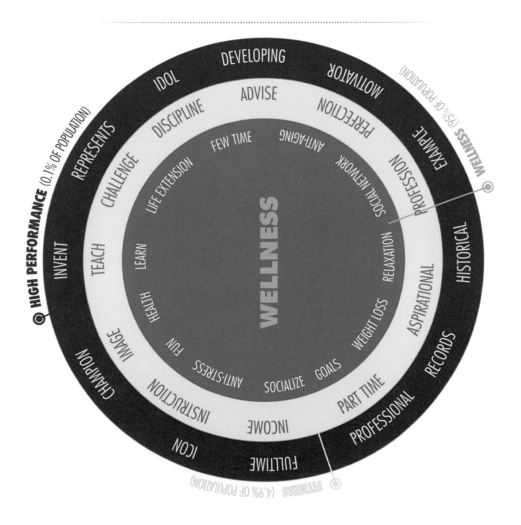

CONTEXT

In the previous chapter, we dealt with many measurements. Let's say now that we have an adult male who has a body fat percentage of 12, with a waist circumference of 88 cm (34.60 inches) and a body mass index of 20. This sounds very good for an apparently Fit Man; I said "apparently" because to evaluate him as a Fit Man in our model, many more measurements should be done. But, you know, these are just numbers! So in this chapter, I would like to talk about the *Qualitative Values* of each segment, to keep getting some more understanding of the differences between them so that we can use them for our benefit.

First of all, from the qualitative point of view, I perceive that the fundamental concepts are as follows: In *High-Performance is Representing Good,* so you concentrate your sessions in competing to *Represent.* In *Fitness is Looking Good,* so your training should pursue mainly a *Good Image.* In *Wellness is Feeling Good,* so your focus should be on physical and mental health so as to *Feel better* and have a *better life.*

What is "representing"? Obviously everybody at the High-Performance wants to win, but you wish to win for many reasons. One of the most important reason is that by winning, everybody—whosoever you or your team is representing—becomes happy because the goal has been attained; however, you have to win with fair play, behaving correctly in and out of the competition itself, dressing properly, and so on, so you do all the necessary endeavors to represent your country, school, university, club, institution, corporation, or yourself in the best possible manner.

What is "looking good"? When you look good, you feel good, right? But that is not the point here; in the last few decades, Fitness has been all about Image, good Shape, models, movie and TV actors, soldiers, and so on. This is great, but I have added to this concept that to be really Fit, you have to be in the right levels outside and inside of your body, including a good performance in factor skills evaluations, not necessarily at the highest level, nor as an athlete, but in a good (or a bit above good) level; here you are really Fit.

What do you understand by "feeling good"? When you win a gold medal, you feel good, or when you go to a beach with a six-pack stomach, you feel good. But here I want to say that you do the amount of physical activity that makes you feel right physically and mentally. You do not really have to run like Usain Bolt or have the perfect buttocks; you just need to do the required physical activity to be healthy so that you put the quantity and intensity of effort required for that, and you feel good with it. Even though I have placed the Sedentary Lifestyle in the bottom levels of Wellness (W1, W2, W3), because we all start there at some point in our lives, you would have noticed that you must move to where the physicians and where WHO have recommended you to be; this is the minimal spot required for any person in the world to have real Wellness, and you will feel good to be here. I have named the Wellness Sweet Spot (see map in chapter 9), but being there, you may want to move to the Fitness levels or maybe become a High-Performer athlete; this is great, but now you know *a Spot that is Sweet for you*, and it is not hard to get there. Just keep reading.

Now, let's take a deeper look at the qualitative values that I think are more related to each segment; however, we may be able to find some of them in any of the three levels.

WELLNESS (W)

Health

According to the World Health Organization (WHO), it is a complete physical, mental, and social Well-Being and not merely the absence of disease or infirmity.

1. Weight Loss: To feel better and to have good health. To be in our right weight is vital; we must diligently watch our weight in the right proportion with our height (see BMI in glossary). Our modern market has become an oversaturated caloric supply of food products and with the lesser-required physical activity of modernity, which has brought obesity and overweight all over. Let's be watchful of what and how much we eat and, of course, our Physical Activity.

2. Anti-Stress: The daily living with its threats causes in us stress, so looking for ways to reduce it brings to us a better living. Meditation, mindfulness, prayer, watching nature or the stars, and so on, may help. But to move our bodies helps us to be relaxed during day and night.

3. Life Extension: To live more years and in better condition could be a good definition of Wellness, so this point is also fundamental for this level. Today, many authors and futurists comment that our lives could be extended easily for more of a hundred years. Therefore, we must take care in conserving our bodies properly.

4. Anti-Aging: To be effective in retarding the effects of aging, it is also an important value of Wellness. Antioxidants, correct diet, skin care, exercise, meditation, learning a new language, and many modern therapies and technologies are coming alongside the technological revolution that we are experimenting, and this is just the beginning.

Fun

To have fun and, beyond that, to enjoy life gives us an awesome feature here. To be happy may soon become one of the most valuable economic variables for the nations. So let's have fun in an active way.

Learning

To know more about our bodies, nutrition, training systems, technology, data, and so on, besides helping us to move up in the levels of Wellness, keeps our minds healthy. Self-awareness, to keep constantly learning about us for better, is an important distinctive.

Socializing

To get to know people in a club, gym, park, or practicing any sport at any place to be accepted by society gives us a healthier manner of socializing much better than 30 years ago when the disco or bar was the rule to meet someone. Today, with the use of social media to reinforce socialization, it could be more fulfilling.

Less Time Required

Not too much time is required daily to get into the Wellness Sweet Spot (see map in chapter 9) compared with the time needed in Fitness and High-Performance.

The WHO (World Health Organization) recommends the following to kids and teenagers from 5 to 17 years old in order to improve cardiorespiratory and muscular "fitness," bone health, and cardiovascular and metabolic health biomarkers:

- Children and youth aged 5–17 should accumulate at least 60 minutes of moderate to intense physical activity daily.

- Amounts of physical activity greater than 60 minutes provide additional health benefits.

- Most of the daily physical activity should be aerobic. Vigorous activities should be incorporated, including those that strengthen muscle and bone, at least three times per week.

For adults aged 18–64:

- Adults aged 18–64 should do at least 150 minutes of moderate aerobic physical activity throughout the week or at least 75 minutes or an equivalent combination of moderate and intense activity.

- Aerobic activity should be performed in bouts of at least 10-minute duration.

- For additional health benefits, adults should increase their moderate aerobic physical activity to 300 minutes per week or engage in 150 minutes of intense aerobic physical activity per week or an equivalent combination of moderate and intense activity.

- Muscle-strengthening activities should be done involving major muscle groups on 2 or more days a week.

For older adults aged 65 and more:

- Older adults should do at least 150 minutes of moderate aerobic physical activity throughout the week or at least 75 minutes of intense aerobic physical activity or an equivalent combination of moderate and intense physical activity.

- Aerobic activity should be performed in bouts of at least 10-minute duration.

- For additional health benefits, older adults should increase their moderate aerobic physical activity to 300 minutes per week or engage in 150 minutes of intense aerobic physical activity per week or an equivalent combination of moderate and intense physical activity.

- Older adults, with poor mobility, should perform physical activity to enhance balance and prevent falls on three or more days per week.

- Muscle-strengthening activities, involving major muscle groups, should be done for two or more days a week.

- When older adults cannot do the recommended amounts of physical activity due to health conditions, they should be as physically active as their abilities and conditions allow.

All these recommendations, as you can see, do not require too much time. *Good Wellness can be done in few hours a week*; between 5 and 10 is what I suggest but always under the supervision of a physician.

Sustainability

To get in a good level of Wellness, it is easier to get and sustain; also, it is cheaper so that more people may be able to feel better reaching this more feasible goal, and the retention levels in clubs could increase. More Wellness all over will bring better people in the industry and society, creating a much better world. *Wellness is more Sustainable than Fitness and High-Performance.*

In the Chapa Wellness Map, for all the reasons that you will be reading in this book, I have placed all these qualitative elements as Wellness, because I have seen that one of the most important reasons of the failure of the current sports model is Perception. Yes! To many people all over our culture, when they listen or see the concept of fitness or sports, some mental barriers come to their minds as something hard to practice and something that they don't have the ability to do, because of past personal failures or just because the media presents people who seem to have come from other worlds, trying to generate aspirational brands and styles. So we must use a different strategy with renewed concepts. We will analyze this theme of Perception in the next chapter.

FITNESS (F)

Image

To look good and to have a good shape is a very attractive motivator to get involved in physical activity, even though not many people get it, and they get discouraged soon. To motivate people is good, and to get motivated for a goal like this is good as well. People can do it by themselves, or they can do it with a personal trainer; this could be better if the resources are available. Reaching these types of hard goals develop character, and that is great too, but when we take a look at World Economic View, we see that this goal is for a small percentage of the global population and that not too many people may be able to reach it. If you want to be at your best, physically speaking, congratulations; it is a great goal, because you will be having the required health elements as well. So . . . *Go for it!*

Perfection

Beyond image, some Fitness enthusiasts may get into a career for perfection that has its advantages (as a fighting courage) and disadvantages (vanity). Muscular symmetry is hard to get but gives a good balanced shape. To have high levels in the factor skills assessments is good for both the body and the mind but requires training and dedication and tends to be a goal for a perfectionist if he or she is not in competition at any sport (performance). To know more and more of a specific training technique could also be considered as perfectionism.

Profession/Teach

Someone who is Fit has already gotten enough knowledge of Wellness and Fitness (according to the Chapa Wellness Map Systematic Approach) to get into that level that is able to teach, to become an instructor or coach (knowing the specifics of a sport) so that with the right certificates of study, this person has already gotten a profession. If this is convenient to him or some people who have reached this high level of physical condition who have another profession may just become some type of advisors for friends or family without charging any fee.

Income

At this point, some already have a profession. Good income could come if you are a personal trainer, instructor, or sports coach. It is time to have some return on investment after many resources given for many years. Obviously, the most important of all possible retribution is the state of having and the knowledge of how to have a body in almost perfect physical condition. Apps and more AI related to Wellness and Fitness, and perhaps robots as personal trainers, will come in the future, but to all of you who train people, remember that the biological experience of having received the benefits of physical activity is a human asset—in other words, the robots just have not learned by living it and by obtaining it firsthand.

Discipline

This may be one of the most important values for Fitness, to focus on executing the programs with a good planned system during many hours a week for many years. It is also a good character trait. Simply, thousands of hours of sweating and pain are required; character, sacrifice, willpower, intelligence, and much more are needed.

Challenge

Trying to be Fit will bring many difficulties, and here are the challenges to overcome. Definitively, this value is required in this yellow circle, and also it is a very good trait to have as part of your personality, someone who can overcome challenges.

Time

More needs to be invested to be Fit than the one required in the Wellness Sweet Spot. I have calculated that between 10 and 20 hours of weekly workouts are required to be classified in this segment. *Fitness is aspirational but requires Time.*

Less Sustainability

To be Fit, as I have defined in this *new Paradigm*, the Chapa Wellness Map, it is harder to get and harder to sustain for almost everybody, so we can congratulate and respect the Fit people. It is a very attractive aspirational goal. We have to be honest that this is a more exclusive level of physical condition or level of sports performance; this is great, but we have to be aware of its pros and cons. Many people who have been Fit have fallen to lower levels of physical condition, and the Chapa Wellness Map defines a more difficult-to-get level of Fitness to have a good separation from the Wellness level, although in the map in chapter 9 we can see that the W10 level is in the frontier with F1.

HIGH-PERFORMANCE (HP)

Representation

To compete for a nation, professional team, university, high school, club, or yourself, doing it at the higher level, having been selected for it in an internal competition or competitions, maybe the Core of this level of physical activity. For not many people are fortunate to have an incredible dream come true, with great rewards and by far well deserved.

Invention

Being at the Top in sports and at the Top of this model, with all the resources of sports medicine, economy (not always), knowledge, time, and so on, in most of the cases exploring new ways to improve, breaking records, creating new technology, creating disruptive technics, and going beyond the limits to win is a fundamental value of this level and one that brings much of the sports development today and has done it in the past too and, I can say, with full of success. But, unfortunately, this does not happen to all, as we have already discussed in this book. Great top professional players and coaches are good innovators—Rafael Nadal's tennis strokes, Bill Walsh's west coast offense, Bill Bowerman's moon shoe, Adidas Telstar's soccer ball, and so on, to name a few.

Science and Technology

To have the best equipment, techniques, nutrition, information, technology, telemetry, knowledge, rehabilitation systems, and so on, are essentials to becoming a champion. Research is key here. To take the human body and mind to the highest levels of performance, new knowledge, and discoveries are necessary.

Professionalism

Even though amateur players are not considered professionals, today I can testify that many of them train like the Pros, and many of the schools' and universities' High-Performance athletes have in their minds to be at some point in their lives a professional player. As we have already discussed, some experts are proposing that the NCAA players should be paid to avoid many controversies.

Championship

Maybe the most important word for good representation is "Win." Great joy and satisfaction come after thousands of hours of hard training, discipline, pain, and sacrifices; great reward is for all of them. Who would be the best champion in all sports of all times would be an interesting question to think about.

Records

Beyond winning, to be the best of all times, to set the new limits, to be the benchmark to imitate, and to beat are key values in this level. I will always remember that perfect 10 that Nadia Comaneci gave us in Montreal in 1976. Beating the best personal mark is always a great motivator for many athletes.

Icon

Media and marketing build together sports icons among High-Performance athletes. That helps to encourage others to follow in their disciplines and, most of the times, set a good example of life. They are global, national, or local icons. *They are Living Brands*, that can generate wealth for the society. Sports industry needs them to operate.

History

The memorable records and feats that an athlete achieves becomes something worth to remember in time. Some of the athletes become legends of a specific sport, country, or institution. To make history in the future is an incentive for many athletes to keep in the fight every day. What do you want to be written in your gravestone would be another interesting question for anybody who is involved in High-Performance.

Full Time

Anyone who applies more than 20 hours a week into intense training is in a full-time level, even though this may be combined with school or work for many. So, compared to Fitness, the person at this level is a full-time athlete. Of course, I am just talking here about hours spent in the gym, track and field, court, mountain, swimming pool, road, and so on, but it is important to remember that these athletes think about their goals, diets, and programs 100 percent of the time, every day of the year, all the years of their active lives as athletes.

Hard to Sustain

Injuries, aging, performance-level decrease, burnout, retirement, and so on, sooner or later come to any player at this level. Here we have the most exclusive segment of this model with its advantages and disadvantages. I want to suggest that many retired athletes must keep a good physical condition to some degree at least. I propose that this is the Wellness Sweet Spot. We have seen many who keep their level almost as when they were athletes. Another thing is that, you see them very Fit in older ages, but I have seen some who look under the recommended levels. High-Performance level is hard to sustain for everybody, including governments, federations, universities, and so on, but it is worthy. The model that I present in this book creates a Virtual Growth Circle that provides resources for all the levels established in the Chapa Wellness Map (see epilogue section letter b) "Wellness Economy").

CHAPTER 6

CHAPA WELLNESS MAP: SPORTS AS THEY ARE PERCEIVED

There are things known and there are things unknown,
and in-between are the doors of perception.

—Aldous Huxley

CHAPA WELLNESS MAP
SPORTS AS THEY ARE PERCEIVED

Which are the PARAMETERS OF PERCEPTION?

A) How easy is to practice in a fun way that activity or sport for any given person?

B) How good should my PHYSICAL CONDITION be to enjoy this sport or activity?

C) Any Activity or Sport presented here could be PERFORMED at WELLNESS, FITNESS or HIGH PERFORMANCE LEVEL.

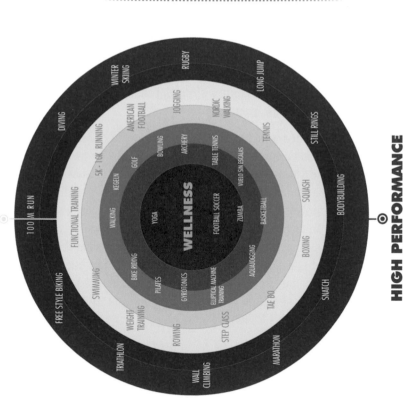

The purpose of this MAP is to present a TOOL that would help to DEVELOP through INNOVATION new SPORTS and PHYSICAL ACTIVITIES that would be PERCEIVED as 'WELLNESS' so that more PEOPLE living SEDENTARY LIVES may find the RIGHT OPTION to START and to MOVE ON in a more ACTIVE and HEALTHIER LIFESTYLE.
Orlando Chapa

"AS THEY ARE PERCEIVED:" WHAT DOES THIS MEAN IN THIS BOOK?

What is perception? One of my Core concepts while writing this book may be this word. What is it? According to *Merriam-Webster's Collegiate Dictionary*, "perception" is derived from "Latin *perceptio-, perceptio* act of perceiving, from *percipere*." It means "a mental image: concept" or a "quick, acute, and intuitive cognition: appreciation" or "a capacity for comprehension." Its synonyms are discernment, insight, wisdom, perceptiveness, perceptivity, sagaciousness, sagacity, and sapience.

My goal for this chapter is to try to systematically classify today's sports in the three segments that are the base of the Chapa Wellness Map; in other words, I am trying to place each sport in the Wellness, Fitness, or High-Performance level based on how the sport may be perceived from any given person according to the level of physical condition required and the difficulty to practice that sport and how easy it is to start playing that sport or to do that activity for a person with minimal physical condition and/or minimal aptitude for sports in general. This could be hard because for some people one sport is easier to practice than the other, and that depends also in the skills required for the sport in particular and the personal abilities of each person, but my purpose to do this is to find out a common denominator or a Set of sports with similar characteristics according to the levels defined in the Chapa Wellness Map.

Why is this very important? Because if we can make some sort of classification, that can help us to understand why some sports are more easy to practice for people who have a Sedentary Lifestyle or in the Chapa Wellness Map Classification in the levels W1, W2, and W3; then we will be in the position to develop more sports belonging to this category. In other words, if you have not yet found the sport or physical activity or exercise technic (as Step, Pilates, Zumba, Squash, etc.), that makes you feel great while you practice it. The probable reason is that it has not been invented yet, so it is possible that you can get involved in developing that concept of activity or sport that has not been created until today. That idea that could come from your own life experience, the concept that you are the only one who can create it. I said to you, go for it!, go invent it! And construct nice roads or whatever you like over this Chapa Wellness Map.

I want to make clear that any sport can be performed at Wellness, Fitness, or High-Performance level. You can have a walk to enjoy some time with your dog in the park (Wellness), or you can walk 30 minutes in the treadmill with 15 percent inclination trying to tone up the buttocks (Fitness), or you can compete representing your country in a 50 km march looking for the Olympic gold medal (High-Performance). I suggest and I am putting the physical activity of Walking in the Wellness Circle because almost everybody in the world can walk, and it is not really difficult to do it, as even babies can do it. So I perceive walking as a Wellness activity, even though it could be performed at Fitness or at High-Performance level as well. So let's go on with this essay to have some sports classified for this book, and I suggest that further research will be necessary in this topic.

WELLNESS (W)-PERCEIVED SPORTS

Walk

It is for me the most representative physical activity for this level as we have seen in the last paragraph. Almost all of us walk, which I do recommend; it is trying to walk a little bit faster and longer every day. For me, it is the easiest way to burn calories, even if I did not have enough sleep or after eating a meal so that I cannot run. Also, when it is about to rain soon, I go out and walk. If you are not in the Wellness Sweet Spot (see map in chapter 9), go out alone, with your partner, son, neighbor, dog, and so on, and do some extra walk; your body will pay it back to you soon.

Bike Riding

Even though it requires some balance to learn to ride a bike, almost anybody can do it; and it is a great exercise and very fun to have a view of the surroundings while riding. Nevertheless, we all know that the Routes Bike Tours involve the highest levels of athletes in their competitions. If you can't ride outside, or you have not learned to do it yet, you can do some activity in a stationary bike at home or get involved in a spinning class at your health club. In Germany, they use the Laufrad, a special bike without pedals for kids under four years old so they can learn to balance and acquire other skills that they require to ride a bike in the future, receiving all the physical benefits while they use their legs to get the impulse directly from the ground.

Yoga

I have seen new yoga practitioners over 65 years old and kids, who learn a Body-Mind activity that helps them to learn how to breath better, get a better posture, balance, increase the blood flow, concentrate, increase self-perception, stretch and relax, have full attention, among many other benefits that are available for everybody in this discipline. To me, yoga is a clear example of a Wellness activity; however, we know yoga masters who can do postures of the highest level of complexity that require many years of hard focused practice. To me, they belong to the group of High-Performance yoga experts.

Soccer

Everybody can kick a soccer ball, maybe not in the right way, but kids, teenagers, adults, and some seniors may be able to play football soccer in one way or another, and I have to say it again that to be a professional in this sport demands a very high athletic condition and lots of natural skills. To see the strength of the game of Cristiano Ronaldo or the quickness of Lionel Messi, it is an expression of the highest level in any professional sport. But to move while kicking a ball trying to score a goal with your family defending in your garden goal is totally a Wellness-perceived sport.

Basketball

In some countries, I have seen basketball street courts in many places. To dribble the ball and to shoot it to the basketball hoop is very fun and demands coordination, balance, and aiming, which involves the mind while counting the steps to bounce the ball before we get into trouble with the referees, trying to pass a defender. And, again, almost everybody has played basketball at some point in their lives, whether in elementary school or junior high. So I believe we have a sport that could fit in the Wellness Green Circle. On the other hand, the NBA and some of the EuroLeague players seem to have come from another planet because of the incredible way they play.

Elliptical Trainer

This activity requires this cardiovascular exercise machine developed by Precor Inc. in 1990. It is an awesome product that could help obese persons to do low-impact aerobic workout in a very easy way but with many benefits for the body; however, kids cannot practice it. Here seniors and people who cannot run because of some type of pain in the back, knee, or ankle can do it. Therefore, for this reason I am placing this activity as a Wellness exercise. Other companies have developed different products that definitively fall in this category but with special features that set them apart, such as the Cybex's Arc Trainer and some equipment of brands like Life Fitness, Technogym, and Octane.

Golf

This sport is one of the most technical sports of all, but it can be played at almost any age because it involves walking around nature, which is good for breathing, relaxing, and stress release; nevertheless, it is expensive almost everywhere. But I have placed it here in perceived-as-Wellness sport, because this sport is a classic one for seniors, who do not practice other sports anymore compared to when they were younger. So I would say that golf is a high-end Wellness sport that makes people feel good without needing a high level of physical condition to play. But I have to point out that to improve requires lots of practice and professional advice, so to become a better player is not easy. Let's say that the ones who know how to play golf can treat it as an easy Wellness activity, and those who do not know can go to the drive range and practice green or mini golf as a Wellness activity alternative, though they will not be receiving the benefit of walking through the 18 holes as the ones that know how to play.

FITNESS (F)-PERCEIVED SPORTS

Fitness being in the middle of these two segments in the Chapa Wellness Map model makes it a little difficult to classify the sports that belong to this Yellow Circle, because it gets squeezed in some way by the other two circles so that the sports that I have placed here could be in some manner perceived as Wellness sometimes or as High-Performance other times. But let's try to get some more understanding of this idea and try to utilize it for our own benefit, whether we want to get involved in more physical activity or are a personal trainer, coach, sport director, entrepreneur, gym or club manager, and so on.

Jogging

If walking is a classical Wellness activity, maybe jogging could be a classical Fitness one, even though anyone may be able to do a short slow run. To make at least 40 minutes of jogging requires some more level of physical condition compared to a 40-minute walk. But jogging is not as demanding as a marathon or as intense as a 100-meter dash, so I keep it in this zone. I could also say that someone who is in the Wellness Sweet Spot level could run one hour or more without any problem. But let's remember that in the Wellness Green Circle exists two lower-level zones; that is where the majority of the global population is.

Boxing

To me it is a great Fitness sport that requires some level of speed, strength, aerobic condition, reaction, footwork, and some technical bases, among other abilities to enjoy it. Even to punch a sack box requires some hand strength so as not to get injured after doing repetitions. In general, this sport helps to develop a muscular body that makes it classical for this Fitness Red Circle in the Chapa Wellness Map. In the professional world, it requires very high levels of physical, technical, and mental abilities and preparation.

Weight Training

Building muscle to have a symmetrical shape makes this activity a classic one for Fitness; however, any person may be able to work out with weights for Wellness purposes, and all Athletes train with weights for strength, power, and so on, so that Weight Training is a great activity for the three segments in this model. However, since, in the last decades, for many people worldwide, it has been done to get a good-looking body, to be Fit, and to have a good Shape, it belongs to the group of Fitness level activities.

Tennis

Getting into the court and playing some games or at least keeping the ball on play over the net without missing requires some level of physical and technical abilities, so I have placed tennis as a basically perceived Fitness Sport. Here we have a good example of a sport that has presented an option to solve its perception as a Fitness Sport, and that is Mini Tennis, a derivative option that requires smaller courts and nets, requires less physical condition and less technical skills compared to Tennis, which makes it great for kids to have fun, be active, and learn. As a Professional Sport, it demands the highest level of physical condition and mental and technical abilities.

Swimming

Despite it being great for relaxing and having a full-body almost-zero-impact workout, it requires the technical skills of knowing how to float and to generate movement with the body extremities. But the experts involved in this discipline have developed alternative techniques on water, such as aqua-jogging, to present a Wellness option for everybody. I believe this Fitness sport has done its work to attend population segments that belong to the lower levels of physical condition. Anyone can go and have some fun in a swimming pool, including kids, burning lots of calories, but to really swim, and enjoy it, much time of practice and learned and developed skills is required. Therefore, I have placed it in the Fitness yellow circle in this model.

HIGH-PERFORMANCE (HP)– PERCEIVED SPORTS

Marathon

I really like this comparison—walking as Wellness, jogging as Fitness, and marathon as High-Performance—to present my idea. These are really different physical activities but, at the same time, are very similar. *I believe this is in the Hearth of the Chapa Wellness Map, "A Systematic Approach to Physical Activity" model.* Nobody can have any doubt that very high physical and mental condition and long preparation are required to run 26.2 miles and to make it in 2:02:574:41.4. You were really born to do it!

Triathlon

A combination of swimming 1500 m, route-cycling 40 km, and running 10k in the Olympic format makes this sport a classical one for me for this level of performance. But if someone who is not a High-Performance athlete wants to do it, I think he or she can do it with the required preparation, being at least at the level of Fitness for participating in smaller-distance Triathlons. I think it is hard that someone at the Wellness level may be able to get in this adventure, unless he or she moves to the next level of intensity of physical activity.

Wall Climbing

Strength in arms, hands, and fingers and explosive strength in legs, balance, and courage to get to the top make wall climbing a High-Performance (HP) Red Circle Sport in this classification that I am presenting here. Kids and beginners can do it in smaller walls with the right protection and instruction to learn and to get Well or Fit to one day become athletes of the wall, some of them, but definitively this is a HP Sport.

Freestyle Biking

Acrobatic performance in a high-performance bike. This is also a sport that belongs, without any doubt, to the most external Red Circle in our new model. It is attractive and extreme, good for media, and a full-time sport that demands many hours of practice and many years to have the control of the Body/Bike duo to do it or at least to not get injured by doing it.

Diving

Strength, balance, coordination, technique, explosive strength, elasticity, concentration, handling pressure, precision, total body control, and so on, make this sport as one that fits perfectly in the High-Performance spot, even though many of us have done a funny jump into the pool at some point in our lives.

ANY POSSIBLE APPLICATION?

A good application of this classification of sports as they are perceived, which I suggest, could be as a *Tool* that would help to develop innovative new sports and physical activities that would be perceived as Wellness so that more people living Sedentary Lives may find the right option to start and to move up into a more Active and Healthier Lifestyle, helping to create the Chain Reaction that could bring and sustain more life. And this is the main reason why I wrote this chapter: to help build the industry. We have millions of adults and much more kids all over the world who have not been involved in some sport or activity yet. Let's disrupt the industry, *let's give a Copernican turn to the model*, let's end the deaths by physical inactivity globally, let's have more years of life and many more of better living for all of us, and let's grow this industry 3× to get the 3.45 percent of the global GDP in 15 years (see letter b) in the epilogue section of this book).

And for those who would think that their sport should be in other level, you may be right. I want to apologize to them and tell them that I wrote all these concepts to construct and not to destroy or hurt; remember that this chapter was all about Perception. Thank you!

To finish, I would like to make it clear that the Wellness level in the Chapa Wellness Map is not just an easy and calm zone or type of activities. Remember that to get to the Wellness Sweet Spot that is right below a Totally Fit Zone, Fitness, we must follow the recommendations of the WHO (World Health Organization), and they require for adults and seniors around 300 minutes a week of moderate or 150 minutes of intense physical activity, mostly aerobic, but also two or three times a week of strengthening exercises involving major group muscles. Also, our assessments must meet the required parameters stated in chapter 8 of this book, the 20 × 20 matrix. Therefore, to do a little extra physical activity, it is better than not doing any at all, but as the body keeps getting in better physical condition, it will be easier for anybody coming from a Sedentary Lifestyle to do more intense physical activity in order to reach the WHO or our physician recommendations.

CHAPTER 7

THE FINANCIAL PARADOX

---

*Your net worth to the world is usually determined by
what remains after your bad habits are subtracted
from your good ones.*

—Benjamin Franklin

CHAPA WELLNES MAP

THE FINANCIAL PARADOX

WHAT DOES IT LOOK LIKE?

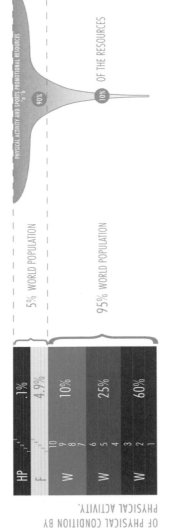

PHYSICAL ACTIVITY AND SPORTS PROMOTIONAL RESOURCES [a] [b]

90%

10% OF THE RESOURCES

5% WORLD POPULATION

95% WORLD POPULATION

HP .1%

F 4.9%

W 10%

W 25%

W 60%

WORLD POPULATION BY LEVEL
OF PHYSICAL CONDITION BY
PHYSICAL ACTIVITY.

WHAT ABOUT THIS WAY TOMORROW?

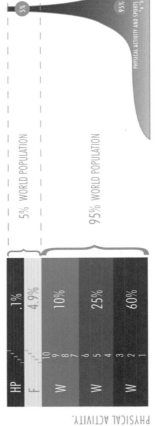

5% OF THE RESOURCES

PHYSICAL ACTIVITY AND SPORTS, PROMOTIONAL RESOURCES [a] [b]

95%

5% WORLD POPULATION

95% WORLD POPULATION

HP .1%

F 4.9%

W 10%

W 25%

W 60%

WORLD POPULATION BY LEVEL
OF PHYSICAL CONDITION BY
PHYSICAL ACTIVITY.

*a According to the CHAPA WELLNESS MAP SEGMENTATION SYSTEM.
*b All the percentage values are assumed for this presentation and will be changed for the real ones during the development of this project.

Orlando Chapa

87

SPORTS IN THE GLOBAL ECONOMY VS. DEATHS FROM PHYSICAL INACTIVITY TODAY

In the introduction of this book, we started to analyze that we have a contradiction in our sports model nowadays; we are having an increase in technology, sports, techniques, sports media presence, professionals' salary, sports events, data, architecture, and so on, in one side and more than 5,000,000 deaths worldwide (World Economic Forum) every year due to a lack of physical activity of a high percentage of the global population (mostly kids) on the other side. We are having a *Paradox* here. But in this chapter, we are going to get deeper into the *Financial Side* of this situation.

In the season 2017–2018, Lionel Messi won just as salary $80,000,000, being the second highest-paid athlete right behind Floyd Mayweather in that year. The Chinese government spent $45,000,000,000 for the Beijing games in 2008, although the estimated amount was $20,000,000,000. The broadcast revenue from Olympic Television Rights of the games held in 2012 in London was $2,600,000,000. The Total Global Sports Industry is calculated between $500,000,000,000 and $1,300,000,000,000 dollars, and the global GDP in the year 2017 was $79,865,480,000,000. This shows that the market share of the Global Sports Industry, including infrastructure construction, sporting goods, licensed products and live sports events, media, and so on, was 1.13 percent of the Global Economy GDP in 2017, if we take the average of the Global Sport Industry information given in the last lines. This is the size of the resources that were dedicated to sports, and we have that physical inactivity is the fourth cause of premature deaths worldwide, among other health problems that come because of lack of physical activity. Doing some numbers from the World Health Organization, I have calculated that in 2012, we had 5.71 percent of global deaths caused by physical inactivity—we had 56,000,000 total deaths worldwide, and 3,200,000 were due to physical inactivity. Just by dividing from the WHO information by 365 days in a year times 24 hours per day times 60 minutes per hour, we have 6.09 people dying per minute due to Physical Inactivity. Remember that this number would be almost the double because other sources indicate that the deaths are above 5,000,000 per year. *A very high cost!*

I think that the total economic resources worldwide destined to the sports industry as related to the World GDP are still small, one of the proofs of all the inactive people we have globally. Remember that we have come from thousands of years, so our bodies used to have Heavy Physical Activity; it is great that with progress and modernity, we don't have to keep doing all that hard work, and robots in the future will help us more and more in doing the heavy stuff, among other things. However, we have to be wise in integrating intelligent Physical Activity in an innovative and disruptive manner in the Workplace, because it is here where we get away from our origins. Here is where I believe we have the Central Point to solve this problem; it is so important to me that I will write a book about it soon.

Work is an economic affair, and our work has become anti-natural to our bodies. This must be corrected to have healthy workplaces, and this is also the reason why we must get into economic matters. We have to learn to manage our health from an economic perspective from the personal all the way to the macroeconomic level. The Sports Industry, which I would like to call now as the Wellness Industry, could grow enormously as a percentage of the GDP, 3 times (3×), to reach more than the 3 percent of the world GDP, as I have calculated, if we do two fundamental things:

1. Reassign the health budget from correction to prevention. This could double the GDP in the Wellness Industry, because even though some may say, "Hey, we are spending the same," I could reply to them, "Yes! But we have reduced deaths by 90 percent as an example, and many, many, many people are living better, longer, and happier." And, you know, people doing these types of activities are less involved in crime, negativity, and other bad habits and are becoming more productive in their jobs. This is good for the person, their families, their companies, their nations, and for the world. So we can conclude that this public policy is wise. I have played with some numbers that I am sharing with you for an example. In Mexico, the Cost of Physical Inactivity is similar to the size of the Mexican Sports Industry, around 0.6 percent of the Mexican GDP, which is $6,000,000,000 us dollars. Here we have a clear example that reassigning resources from Cost to Investment, from Correction to Prevention, we could double the size of a very positive industry to the society while mitigating the harmful effects of the situation that we are facing today. Of course, this transition may take a few years, but this is a Win-Win scenario that we are creating. *Here we have doubled the GDP of the industry from the initial number, 1.13 percent, to a very feasible 2.26 percent.* This resource reallocation must come from governments in deep collaboration with the companies that may have interest in; just political will and coordination is required.

Adding this number to the initial global GDP that we had, we get:

1.13 + 1.13 = 2.26% of the global GDP in the World Wellness by the Physical Activity Industry
2.26% x $79,865,480,000,000 = $1,804,000,000,000 (2017)

2.   As more and more people get initiated in Physical Activity, leaving their deadly lifestyle, many will demand new activities and products; in other words, they will move up in the levels of the Chapa Wellness Map. If we listen to their needs and guide them with new approaches to keep discovering their bodies as a healthy, beautiful, and incredible asset, which the robots and AI don't have, *I see that the market could double* by this reason also, as more people get in the higher levels of Wellness, Fitness, and High Performance. We can have here another 1.13 percent.

Adding both numbers to the initial GDP that we had, we get:

1.13 + 1.13 + 1.13 = 3.39% of the global GDP in the Wellness by the Physical Activity Industry
3.39% x $79,865,480,000,000 = $2,707,439,772,000 (2017)

We will see this subject again in the epilogue section of this book.

CURRENT MODEL

From the data mentioned earlier, we can see that 1.13 percent of the Global GDP dedicated to sports is not enough to reduce the Cost of Physical Inactivity (see map in chapter 1). But we also have another problem coming from the current sports model: utilizing the Chapa Wellness Map segmentation helps us to see more clearly, and we have given too much emphasis to the High-Performance and the Fitness levels and not enough attention to Wellness where we have probably 95 percent of the world population, with the assessments given in this book (see map in chapter 8).

Let's assume that 0.10 percent of the global population is in the High-Performance level and that 4.90 percent is in the Fitness level. This gives us a total of 5.0 percent, adding High-Performance and Fitness. Let's say as I perceived it that we have 90 percent of the promotional resources destined to these two segments, because we can see it that way in our daily lives (TV sports professionals, sports infrastructure investment as sponsored stadiums, good-looking Fit bodies in TV Programs and Fitness Products Advertisings, infomercials, etc.), and we do not see too much promotion directed to the 95 percent of the people left. The Wellness Green Circle promotes to reduce weight, waist size, fat percentage, and aerobic condition; to correct levels on blood chemistry; to age better; to take sports as medicine; and mindfulness—or Wellness in general, where we may be having just 10.0 percent of the sports promotional global budget. Most of this promotion is done by governments, as the Mexican program "Check you, Measure you, Move" and some other is done by infomercials, which, nevertheless, recommend weight reduction among other benefits of exercise. Most of the time they just sell Miracle Products, products that cannot satisfy the offered claims when the consumer has acquired them. We can see here clearly that something is wrong; we are investing the promotional resources upside down.

What do we have here? What is the message to all the inactive and scarcely active people of the world? Be a spectator; sit; have chicken wings, pizza, and beer; and enjoy the spectacle, like in those days in the Roman Coliseum; but remember that in those days people used to do much more Physical Activity to make their living. To be just a spectator is not bad once a week, but all the media is presenting us athletes very busy competing, not recommending us why to get active; not even the TV commentators do it. We don´t see common people like us in the media share the benefits of Wellness to us, passivity prevails.

We have 80 percent of inactive kids worldwide. Why? It was assumed that kids would follow and imitate their star athletes, but they have not done it; kids prefer to play the video game of that sport in particular or any other video game, a passive video game, and parents are busy working or too tired from the hard work at office during weekdays when they return home; therefore, nowadays, kids are fat.

I just want to be critical here so that we can construct new options as you have seen during this book. I want to recognize once again that the Sports Industry has accomplished many good things for our society, but I really think we can do much better for the benefit of many, mainly for those who are reading these lines.

NEW MODEL

What could happen if we may be able to do the inverse? What if we invest 95 percent of the global promotional resources for Sports and Physical Activity into Wellness? We may thus reach the 95 percent of the population, and the rest 5 percent of the resources to the 5 percent of the people. By this I am not saying that we should reduce the investment in High-Performance and Fitness activities but that we should invest in all kind of new resources, such as ideas, community work, public policy, innovation, time, synergies, social networks, IT, AI, Industry 4.0, and many other resources besides money, to get this *Paradigm Shift* that could help us to get rid of those more than 5,000,000 deaths every year.

If we analyze these numbers deeper, we can get a 28 × factor (28 times factor), because today we have a 9 to 1 ratio:

High-Performance + Fitness = 90% of the promotional resources
Wellness receiving just 10% of the promotional resources

THE **CHAPA WELLNESS MAP**

And after analyzing the situation with the Green Wellness at the center of the model (by this I am trying to say that we all must give priority to Wellness)—Chapa Wellness Map—we may be able to get in the future the Paradigm Shift, a Cultural Change, trying to solve the Paradox, getting a more reasonable 19 to 1 Ratio:

Wellness = 95% of the promotional resources
High Performance + Fitness = 5% of the promotional resources

To match the population percentages, here we have a factor of 9 (from the 9 to 1 as it is today) + a factor of 19 (from the 19 to 1 that should be) = 28 times factor. This means we are having a deficit of 28 TIMES (28×) of promotional resources not applied to the Wellness Circle or Population Segment., Here we have all the sedentary people presenting the risk factors that are generating diseases related to physical inactivity, and here is the place where more than 5,000,000 people die every year because they don´t meet the recommended Physical Activity by the WHO. I believe this could end the Killing Lifestyle of Physical Inactivity that we are having today. Sounds like a dream but why not change? Note: These are estimated numbers to illustrate the model.

Visualize the following scenarios:

Scenario 1: You are watching your favorite football team, and the TV commentator tells all the audience, "For every goal that your team scores, you will do 10 push-ups, and for every goal of the opposite team, you will do 10 sit-ups." In the halftime of the same game, Adidas-sponsored section offers 50 soccer balls to the first 50 videos sent to the X, Y, or Z digital address, from anyone who does 20 squats with hands on the back of the neck.

Scenario 2: Cristiano Ronaldo has just made another hat trick. During the interview at the end of the game, he just tells all the audience that it is vital to activate, and for this, he teaches how to get the BMI, explaining that this is a very important measure to keep healthy and to have a better life and that with sports like football, walking, or bike-riding with a balanced diet, the correct levels of BMI can be achieved.

Scenario 3: The Allianz stadium management team in Munich, Germany, has placed all over the stadium a *Wellness Spot*, where kids and adults can do some zigzags, do small runs avoiding cones, jump over a painted ladder, and walk up and down in some special stairs that tells you how many you have done and how many you must do to have a good fast workout. Outside the restrooms, men and women can find a belt for the waist, which you cannot fasten if your don't have 90 cm as a man or 80 cm as a woman. Those who can fasten will have a good discount for the ticket of next game. These and more activities are constantly advertised at loud in the stadium's local sound.

Scenario 4: Rafael Nadal, after winning another match during his interview, gets a quick ultrasound test to let the TV and stadium audience know his body fat percentage, telling them that this is an important test to be an athlete or simply a good thing to enjoy a better and longer life, also telling everybody that playing tennis helps to get the recommended levels of fat percentage by the physicians.

Scenario 5: The most respected coach of the NFL has started in his Facebook page a complete section to help everybody who wants to Be Active and give them many tips on how to do it. With a football, anyone can get some fun and improve many skill factors while reducing some weight for those who need it.

Scenario 6: An elementary school, being aware of the inactivity of their students, has implemented that every two hour of classes, the kids must do 10 minutes of physical activity, including stretching, strength exercise using their own bodyweight, and some walking. At the end of each *Wellness Break*, the teacher gives them a 3-minute verbal exposition of the importance of having a healthy diet to be a better student and to have a healthier and better future.

As you can see, all these cases don't require large amounts of financial resources; they just need creativity and imagination, and just using the free spaces, normal interview time, social media, and so on, the invitation for a more active lifestyle can be easily done but requires the action of many.

PART II

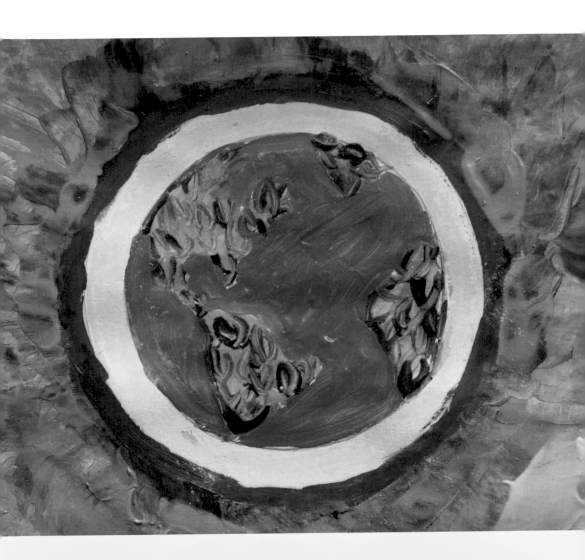

CHAPTER 8

MATRIX 20 × 20

As far as the laws of mathematics refer to reality, they are not certain, and as far as they are certain, they do not refer to reality.

—Albert Einstein

MATRIX 20X20

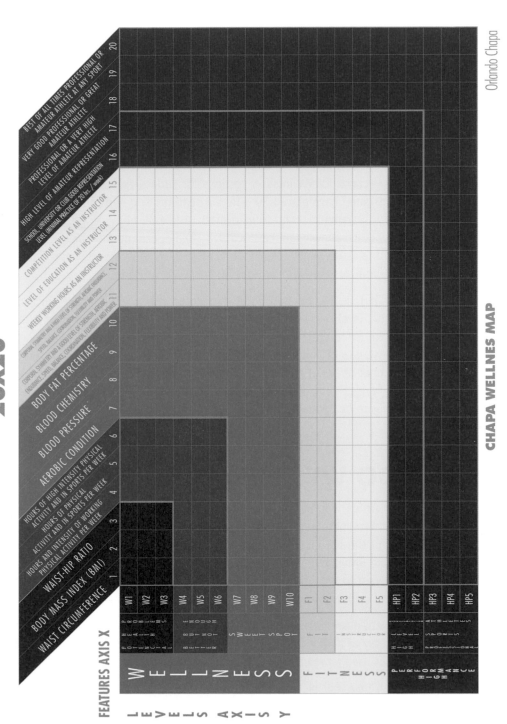

Orlando Chapa

CHAPA WELLNES MAP

97

WHAT IS THE MATRIX 20 × 20?

Basically it is a chart that I developed so we can see the Chapa Wellness Map's 20 divisions in a very practical way, the same that are in the Concentric Circles Model (see map in chapter 4), that are constituted by 10 sections for Wellness (from W1 to W10), 5 sections for Fitness (from F1 to F5), and 5 sections for High-Performance (from HP1 to HP5). All these are in the vertical column or AXIS Y, thinking about the Cartesian Plane. In the opposite column, the horizontal or AXIS X, we have 20 sections also divided in the same 10 sections for Wellness, 5 sections for Fitness, and 5 sections for High-Performance, but here I have placed 20 different features or group of features, one for each section in a systematic progression related to health, physical activity, physical condition, skill factors, knowledge, certifications, and sports performance level. After getting to know the assessments of the interested person, *he or she will know his or her Wellness Level as it is classified in the Chapa Wellness Map System.*

Getting into the details, we are starting at the center with a very inactive child as an example of the W1 level (Wellness level 1), moving all the way up to the most external and final level, the HP level 5 (High Performance level 5), where we will be having the best sport professionals or amateurs of all times at their sport or activity, like Michael Jordan in basketball or Roger Federer in tennis. The way in which we will obtain the results for these levels will be seeing later on during this chapter, where we will analyze closer the *Features to be Assessed* in the AXIS X or horizontal section.

WHY DO WE NEED IT?

To make things easier, it is by far more practical for almost everybody to say "I am now in W9 level" (Wellness level 9) than to say "I am an adult man, 51 years old, who got rid of most of the risky health factors linked to physical inactivity, such as being overweight (where BMI>24.9); doing less than five hours a week of moderate physical activity; having waist-to-hip ratio bigger than .90, body fat percentage as 26, high levels of LDL cholesterol, and high levels of triglycerides; and so on."

So this person, with a combination of one letter and one number W9 in this case, has a number that is easy to handle and remember and which contains all that data, and all this data could be used for many who look for a healthier and happier society.

This system with time will be very practical, because it will concentrate on a lot of information about us, and when we get it digitalized, we will be able to reach millions of people worldwide. However, the most important thing is that you start to know your level and move as soon as possible to the recommended levels or to a higher one, the one that you may like to have as your personal objective so as to get into the Fitness Zone because you want to win that squash tournament in your office or look incredible at the beach.

WHO CAN USE IT?

- Anyone interested in improving his or her health, image, sports performance, and so on, for a better, longer, and happier life, with a very useful tool. Use this Matrix to know more about yourself by watching how your physical activity and diet change many of these variables. You have two options: get your Wellness Level, or if you want to know how it is constituted, you can see all the 20 × 20 Matrix chart filled with your data to have a detailed outlook.

- Personal trainers, coaches, sports directors, club managers, and so on, in gyms, clubs, spas, and so on, can motivate members with a compact and visual tool to show them where they are and to help them accomplish their goals. You can help them to get to know their Wellness Level and guide them to move up to the more convenient ones, seeing clearly all the elements involved to be taken in consideration for the assessment.

- Human resource managers, corporate wellness managers, and so on, to reduce presenteeism, absenteeism, reduce DALYs, improve productivity, improve workplace environment, etc.. They can encourage their employees to learn more about all the elements that are involved in getting into the optimal Wellness Levels and to reach them in an easy, practical way.

- Product managers, marketing managers, entrepreneurs, and so forth, to develop strategies for specific market targets. They can work with both columns, with the Wellness Levels or with the elements that will give us the Level. New products, services, campaigns, and so on, can be developed to change our culture into a healthier one, which is good for everybody.

- Researchers, teachers, scientists, and so on, to keep increasing the knowledge in these topics, to develop new theory and technologies for the health of the human body and for this industry, and to be more precise and updated in all Wellness-related data.

- Technologists and futurists, like Gerd Leonhard, with all the trends of the Fourth Industrial Revolution and with his growing concepts of digitization, mobilization, screenification, disintermediation, decentralization, automation, intelligization, virtualization, anticipation, and robotization. Many opportunities are present to develop disruptive ideas utilizing this Wellness Matrix for the benefit of many in need.

- Economist, to use the available resources in a more sustainable way in a wiser manner. The Wellness Economy is just starting to be understood and appreciated.

- Public policy makers and governments can utilize all this information to solve this world's social and health problem. Local, national, and global information could be obtained so that they can act in a more accurate manner in this theme.

- Health institutions, physicians, and so on, for their prevention programs. We are creating user-friendly applications so that their patients and interested people can understand it better and can be motivated to get the correct levels.

- NGOs, social entrepreneurs, social programs and so forth can have more tools to help the public and the private sector to end this Global Pandemic. We have seen at the FIBO trade show in Cologne Germany organizations as *Europeactive*, that promotes that *more people* all over Europe can be *more active, more often*; and the *German program Integration Durch Sport*, that looks that immigrants in Germany can be more integrated in their society, as some from their staff have said, "Der Sport bringt Bewegung in die Integration" (Sport brings Movement into Integration); so we have here another element that we hadn't considered before.

In the next sections, we will have a closer description of both columns, AXIS Y and AXIS X, trying to get some more understanding of this 20 × 20 Matrix, which will be helping in many ways all the people who are physically inactive and active and to all those who, like me, are involved in this fascinating industry.

LEVELS 20 / AXIS Y (VERTICAL SECTION)

Wellness / W / Center Green Circle / AXIS Y

I have subdivided this section into three smaller ones (also see the map in this chapter).

1. POTENTIAL HEALTH PROBLEMS ZONE RELATED TO THE LACK OF PHYSICAL ACTIVITY—SEDENTARY LIFESTYLE LEVEL

In this first section, we have the W1, W2, and W3 levels, where we have the *Sedentary Lifestyle segment that has to be activated*, because the people who fall in this category have the highest risk of getting a disease related to physical inactivity. An example of people in this segment could be a 39-year-old lady who may be working part time in an office, has three kids, and does not have apparently any time to do physical activity or exercise apart from taking care of the kids and doing the usual activity at home and at the office; moreover, she does not eat very healthy, so she is obese, with a big belly, and she gets exhausted after climbing just a few steps on the stairs. This is the real situation of many adults living in the cities all over the world. Awareness of the need to allocate resources, mostly time and effort to go and walk and to move more for our own benefit is required. We will have plenty of personal benefits, family benefits, and social benefits if we work hard to support the people who are in the *first section*. I think we can do it with some imagination and with all the technological resources available.

2. BETTER BUT NOT ENOUGH

In this *second section*, I am presenting the next three levels of Wellness—W4, W5, and W6—where people have already started to move more, but the amount of time given with the combination of intensity is *Better but not Enough* to obtain the desired results, like getting into the Wellness Sweet Spot. Motivation to start a good physical activity program and to reach the goal desired has to be promoted; these people may be half of the way far off the place where they will have all the benefits of having significantly reduced the risk of health problems related to physical inactivity. For example, an office worker plays three hours of tennis on weekends and goes to take a one-hour slow walk twice a week. He is doing better but not enough. He has to increase his physical activity from four to five or more days a week and has to look for a more complete exercise program, watching his diet and checking his BMI (see Glossary), waist-hip ratio, aerobic condition, blood chemistry, and so on, to get into the Wellness Sweet Spot.

3. THE WELLNESS SWEET SPOT LEVEL

This third section is the key for this model, the Wellness Sweet Spot of the Chapa Wellness Map, where I have placed the next four levels of Wellness—W7, W8, W9, and W10. It is here where we could have the Paradigm Shift that I am proposing so that people of the world can have a more *sustainable and easier-to-reach zone* for their level of physical condition (see map in chapter 9). Furthermore, among other modern options, they can utilize all the information technology tools that are coming into our smartphones day by day, cheaper and cheaper, so that they may be able to know they are getting there in a *healthier spot*, where they have reduced their risk of diseases and so feel better in body and mind. This has happened because they have increased the weekly time, intensity, and variety of physical activity and/or sports and have been doing it for longer periods of time, involving more months of activity sessions and keeping a healthy diet. And even though they are not 100 percent Fit, as we have defined in this book, they have reached this great level of Wellness by having a physically active and healthier lifestyle.

As an example, we may have here someone already exercising six hours a week divided into five or six days, with a good combination of strength, aerobic condition, flexibility, mobility, and coordination workouts or with a sport that involves all or many of these features; having a good balanced diet; and depending on many other factors as his initial physical condition for, let's say, more than six months. Sounds hard, but it is not; *the Chapa Wellness Map can help you get to this Sweet Spot,* just going step by step and letting your body get better and better. The different ascendant levels of each category will help you to do that; but remember that *something is better than nothing.*

Fitness / F / Middle Yellow Circle / AXIS Y

I have subdivided this Fitness Yellow Circle in two sections, where the First Section has the first two levels of Fitness (F1 and F2), and the Second Section has the next three levels (F3, F4, and F5).

1. FIT LEVEL

In the first two levels of Fitness, we need the levels of biometry and the skill factors to be correct and corporal symmetry to be obvious so that people notice that you are Fit. So here anyone who is in F1 or F2 levels has all the measurements of biometry correct (see AXIS X, which follows), such as the waist circumference; body mass index; waist-hip ratio; hours and intensity of labor and training; aerobic condition; blood pressure; blood chemistry and body fat percentage; visible body symmetry; and from good to high level of strength, endurance, speed, balance, coordination, elasticity, and power. The only difference between F1 and F2 is that in F1 level, a person has a Good level in the seven skill factors mentioned earlier and in the F2 level, the person has a High level.

Here the qualitative values of image, shape, and perfection are present, and *the Key concept of Looking Good is exalted.* All the health values are implicit here as well because to be in these first two Fitness levels, you must have all the features of Wellness correct. *Many people that want to perform better at any sport without being a High-Performance Athlete must reach F1 or F2 to get the desired Performance.*

2. INSTRUCTOR LEVEL

We are moving into the Instruction and Profession qualitative values. Someone who is in this Fitness level, in this second section that includes F3, F4, and F5 levels, is classified to be here because he or she has the knowledge of how to get here. He or she can teach by being a Personal Trainer, Instructor, or Coach, paid or not paid; also, this person probably has already started to get deeper in education by attending courses in order to become a

Certificated Instructor or a Certificated Personal Trainer, and some of them have started to Compete—not as a High-Performance athlete yet, but he or she is diverging to the outer Red Circle, training to win in competitions in a more serious way compared with someone in the Wellness Level that sometimes could compete but more to socialize than to really break his hearth to win.

Some instructors do not keep 100 percent Fit all the time. Fitness level is hard to get and sustain, so we will use double classification system for people above F2 (Fitness 2), like some master trainer who has a high level of knowledge in training technics and has many certificates as an instructor, who is definitively an F4 (Fitness 4), but, let's say, after an injury, he is not Fit. So this teacher may be classified as an F4 (W9), Fitness 4 (Wellness 9), to notice that he has a good classification as an instructor but that at certain moment he is not 100 percent Fit, but he remains in a very good Wellness Level, the W9, in The Sweet Spot, because he keeps himself physically active enough with a healthy diet.

High-Performance / HP / Outer Red Circle / AXIS Y

Finally, we are going to see a little bit deeper the subdivisions that I am presenting for this third level. I am dividing this zone in two sections.

1. GOOD AND HIGH LEVEL OF AMATEUR REPRESENTATION

We have here the levels HP1 and HP2 (HP for High-Performance), where we have just amateur athletes from clubs, academies, schools, universities, companies, sponsors teams, self-representation, and so on, who train at a High Level of Intensity for more than 20 hours a week, with the aim of *Representing* through competition their institutions, schools, teams, companies, brands, themselves, etc.. They have specialized coaches, high-quality facilities in many cases (but there are exemptions), good programs, specialized nutrition, great training machines, sport science applied, and so forth, but even though they are full-time athletes, they combine it with other activities, such as school, work, family, and so on. But some of them are already becoming, or will soon become, Professionals in their respective sport or activity.

2. PROFESSIONALS AND VERY HIGH LEVEL OR MORE AMATEUR SPORTS ATHLETES

Now paid Professionals have appeared—HP3, HP4, and HP5; they are Full-Time Athletes, looking to be the best of their countries, world, and history. However, we also have here unpaid athletes at the higher level of competition as some of the Top Universities and National Olympic Athletes, who, in many nations, do not get paid, but in some way they get supported by governments, foundations, and/or sponsors. The HP3 level (High-

Performance 3), I could say, is any professional player or a good one of any professional team or one of a very good university, school, city, or state. The HP4 (High Performance 4) is already a very good professional athlete or a great amateur athlete striving with all his heart to improve. An HP5 (High-Performance 5) is The Best-of-all-Times Professional or Amateur athlete of his discipline or sport. Here we have the Champion, the Icons, almost-impossible-to-break Record holders, who make, and have made, History, where they use all the Sport Science available, and they Invent in many ways for the benefit of all the sports and physical activity. These are the ones who have made millions of dollars in their sport in the last few decades.

Nevertheless, we have all the bad side effects that we have already discussed in Chapter 3. They could be reversed in an important manner giving more attention to the Wellness Green Circle in the Model that I present in this book.

Features to Be Assessed 20 / Horizontal Section / AXIS X

Now we have the Features to be Assessed to obtain the 20 levels of classification given in the previous paragraphs. I am presenting a 20 × 20 Matrix system, 20 levels × 20 features. This is going to be done by answering a few questions for Preliminary Level (see letter *a) Do you want to know your Wellness Level? Get it now!* in the Special Topics section of this book) and after, with different tests in each person who may have the interest to know his or her Precise Level of Wellness by Physical Activity.

For Wellness / W / Measurement / Features 1 to 10 / AXIS X (see map in this chapter)

We will be using the next measurements to classify the Wellness Levels; therefore, I have used the same subdivisions and colors as used in the Levels AXIS Y.

1. FIRST SECTION

Waist Circumference, Body Mass index (BMI), and Waist-Hip Ratio. I have placed them first because they are easy to understand and easy to measure so that people may be able to start increasing their Wellness rating by focusing in getting these three elements to the correct levels at first. The corporal weight will be used to get the BMI (weight in kilograms / height in meters squared) and the resultant number mostly between 18.5 and 24.9 to be in the correct level. The recommended Waist Circumference must be under 94 cm (37 inches) for adult men and under 80 cm (31.50 inches) for adult women. The

Waist-Hip Ratio is the proportion that we get by dividing the waist size by the hip size; the recommendation of the WHO is that the ratio must be under 0.90 for adult men and under 0.85 for adult women.

2. SECOND SECTION

Now, we are going to evaluate Hours and Intensity of Working Physical Activity per Week (at the workplace or at home), Hours Spent for Physical Activity and Sports per Week, and Hours Spent in High-Intensity Physical Activity and Sports per Week that correspond to the levels W4, W5, and W6 in the other column. In the Wellness level, we will have people who have done from 0 to less than 10 hours per week of physical activity and/or sports, besides all the activity at their jobs.

The assessment of these first two sections can be done in a few minutes with a tape measure and a weighing machine (which many people have or are easy to get) to obtain the measurements and answering the questions of the second section, which can be done in a minute. You can get your preliminary Wellness Level now with this information (see letter a) in the Special Topics section.

3. THIRD SECTION

That was made to match from W7, W8, W9, and W10 in the Levels side, AXIS Y. I am incorporating to measure Aerobic Condition, Blood Pressure, Blood Chemistry and Body Fat Percentage; these values are a little bit harder to obtain, because they need other types of instruments and require more time as is the case with the blood chemistry test. The body fat percentage and blood pressure require good instruments, even though there are many commercial ones not very accurate. The Aerobic Condition—a good aerobic condition—is the state where the heart and lungs can pump blood more efficiently, allowing more oxygen to be delivered to the muscles and organs; a good test is to run or jog 2.415 kilometers (1.5 miles) and see how much time is required. The time in this test besides the aerobic condition depends also in sex and age. *Always remember to check with your doctor before getting into any more demanding physical activity or test.* The Blood Pressure is the measurement of the pressure of the blood in the artery; an optimal blood pressure is a reading under 120/80 mmHg, but your physician will advise you what is your ideal blood pressure. Blood Chemistry is a test done on a sample of blood to measure the amount of certain substances in the body. For our classification, we will consider a cholesterol test, which will measure the amount of cholesterol and triglycerides in the blood, and a blood glucose test that will measure the concentration of glucose in the blood. The Body Fat Percentage is the amount of fat contained in the body; it is measured as a percentage, and the recommended levels vary with sex and age.

There are many ways to obtain it, but any nutritionist or personal trainer may help you to get this measurement.

Whosoever gets good results in these first 10 tests will be in the higher levels of The Wellness Sweet Spot for sure and very close to the Fitness Circle. So now, we are going to measure some skill factors and new parameters that belong to the Fitness Level.

For Fitness / F / Measurement / Features 11 to 15 / AXIS X

As I did it in the first 10 features of the horizontal column or AXIS X that matched the first 10 levels of Wellness of the vertical column or AXIS Y, these five new characteristics or groups of characteristics of the horizontal column or AXIS X now correspond to measure the five Fitness Levels in the AXIS Y.

We have two sections here.

1. FIRST SECTION

Here we have two groups of features to be assessed and are presented to match with F1 and F2. For F1 we are going to measure Corporal Symmetry and a Good level of Strength, Aerobic Endurance, Speed, Balance, Coordination, Flexibility, and Power. For F2 we are going to measure the same, except for a small change; in that, instead of a Good Level of these Skill Factors, a High Level is required, without getting into the High Performance Levels.

- With Corporal Symmetry, I refer to an evenly distributed muscle mass that is symmetrically pleasing, so here we have *the key qualitative value of Fitness for me. You look good!*

- Strength can be defined as the maximum force a muscle or a group of muscles can apply against a resistance; the one repetition maximum weight is a good example of a test to measure what is the maximum weight a person can lift in one repetition of a specific exercise.

- Aerobic Endurance is the ability of the heart and lungs to work for a long period of time; an example is the Harvard step or the Cooper test (12-minute run).

- Speed is how quickly a person can move. A 50-meter run or, as in the NFL, the 40-yard run are good examples of speed tests.

- Balance is the ability to hold the body in a position without moving or the ability to keep the equilibrium while moving. Keeping the equilibrium with one leg is a good example of test for this skill factor.

- Coordination is the ability to use two or more parts of the body at the same time under control. The wall toss test could be used here.

- Flexibility is the capacity of a joint or muscle to move through its full range of motion. We have the sit-and-reach test as a good option.

- Power or Explosive Strength is the combination of using strength and speed at the same time. The vertical jump is a classical test for this skill.

I want to highlight that people who compete in sports events such as tournaments, competitions, matches, contests, and so on, and who are not in the High-Performance Level, train themselves to Perform better at any sport or activity; they will probably fall in the F1 or F2 category because of the hours invested in training and competition and because of their results in all the assessments. Our Fitness Level (this book/model concept of Fitness) is a good level for Sports Performance, plus the required specific sports abilities.

There is a very important thing here that I need to explain. As the F2 Level (Fitness 2 Level) is the highest Rank in this classification system related to biometry, skill factors, time, and intensity of physical activity of anyone who is not an athlete, we could say that after 10 levels of Wellness, plus 2 levels of Fitness, 12 levels in total, we are covered; in other words, the 12th level, F2, is the maximum level possible related to the physical condition of someone who is not an athlete.

The next eight levels that we will see are related to Profession and Professionals concepts, which, I see, are for Fitness Instructors that could be also Instructors for Wellness as well and with High-Performance Athletes.

2. SECOND SECTION

We will have three features to measure; they are Weekly Working Hours as an Instructor, which is related to F3 in the levels of AXIS Y; Level of Education as an Instructor, which corresponds with the F4 Fitness level; and Competition Level as an Instructor, which intersects the F5 level in the AXIS Y. We have to be aware that we are starting to measure Competition, which is a fundamental concept for High-Performance-related features.

So here we are not measuring any more the body internally or externally; we are now considering Professional activities, Curriculum, and some Competition, and as we can see, the level of involvement in physical activity keeps growing higher and higher.

For High-Performance / HP / Measurement /Features 16 to 20 / AXIS X

Now we will take a look at the last five characteristics to be evaluated, the ones that will help us to know who gets the higher levels, the High-Performance ones. I am dividing it in two sections.

1. FIRST SECTION

We have the 16th and 17th features that we will evaluate. For the 16th that corresponds to HP1 (High-Performance Level 1), consider if this person is someone who belongs to a School, Academy, University, or Club with a Good Level of Representation in competitions with minimal practice of 20 hours per week or more of a very good intensity of physical activity, corresponding to HP1 in the AXIS Y. As the 17th characteristic, we will assess if this is an athlete with a High Level of Amateur Representation(meaning one who has outstanding performances in local or state competitions), that intersects HP2 in the High-Performance Levels. In this section, we deal mostly with Amateur athletes.

2. SECOND SECTION

This is the final one, and here we have the Professionals and the Higher Levels of Amateur players or competitors. So in the 18th feature to be measured, the key question is if he or she is a Professional or a very High-Level Amateur Athlete corresponding to HP3 (High-Performance 3). For the 19th, we have someone who classifies as a very Good Professional or a Great Amateur Athlete and matches with HP4 (High-Performance level 4). Finally, we have the *Dream Place for many people* who have played a sport as a kid or a teenager, trying to become as that TV Sport Star someday. Here we have this important 20th question to be answered, that very few could answer Yes. The questions is, "Are you one of the BEST OF ALL TIMES PROFESSIONAL OR AN AMATEUR ATHLETE AT ANY SPORT OR ATHLETIC COMPETITION?" If someone answers with a Yes, he or she will be having the highest possible score—HP5, (High-Performance 5). After this, I don't have anything left to say about this athlete than to just show my highest admiration and respect for him or her.

With the objective of bringing to ZERO the number of deaths due to Physical Inactivity, we need to know the level of Physical Activity done by the people. Once we know the level of one person, we could know the level of a district, then of a country, and then of more countries, and finally the world so as to be in the World Classification System of the Levels of Wellness by Physical Activity (see map in chapter 10).

Now you have a general idea of the levels and the assessments that we will be using to know your Level of Wellness by Physical Activity, according to the Chapa Wellness Map. If you want to know your Preliminary Level, you will be able to do it in less than 3 minutes right now, if you go to the Special Topics section of this book (letter a) "Do you want to know your Wellness Level? Get it now!". Get your level, and Move Up to the one that you most desire. Be Active, Be Well, Be Alive!

CHAPTER 9

....

THE WELLNESS SWEET SPOT

....

You are never too old to set another goal or to dream a new dream.

—C. S. Lewis

THE WELLNESS SWEET SPOT

BE ACTIVE, BE WELLNESS, BE ALIVE

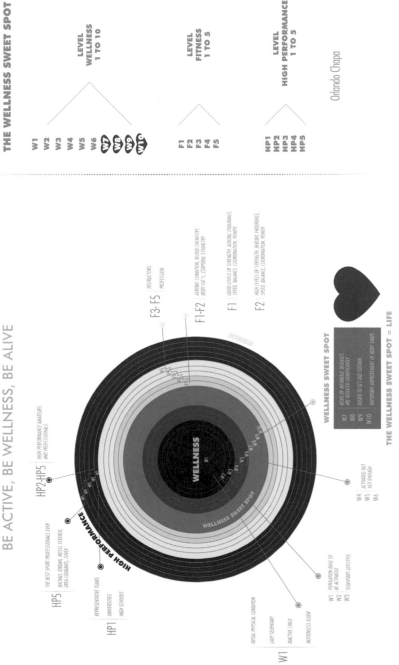

THE WELLNESS SWEET SPOT

W1
W2
W3
W4
W5
W6

LEVEL
WELLNESS
1 TO 10

F1
F2
F3
F4
F5

LEVEL
FITNESS
1 TO 5

HP1
HP2
HP3
HP4
HP5

LEVEL
HIGH PERFORMANCE
1 TO 5

Orlando Chapa

WHY DEVELOP A WELLNESS SWEET SPOT?

While playing tennis in the 1980s as a teenager, I remember some specialized magazines like *World Tennis* that used to make recommendations for the new technology rackets, pointing out how big and where the Sweet Spot was in a new model developed for any famous brand, such as Prince, Wilson, Head, Dunlop, Rossignol, ProKennex, Puma, Yonex, Völkl, Kneissl, and so on. In those days, I was learning the English language, among many other things, and I do not remember exactly how it happened, but while I was starting to build this model, I chose this phrase, The Sweet Spot, to use it in the Chapa Wellness Map, adding it to the new concept of Wellness that I was meticulously thinking. I want to share with you that this phrase came to my mind the first time from tennis, referring to that special zone where you should hit the tennis ball to have the best shots.

So, for me, this chapter is the Key for the Chapa Wellness Map model, because it is where I think owners of fitness centers may be able to get the highest scores in member retention, thereby minimizing the attrition of gyms, clubs, and spas. *Moreover, people who are involved in physical activity may know a more reachable objective and one of a very high value: Life.* From the beginning of any Fitness Program—although now we could say Wellness Program— physically active people could look for a goal easier to reach and sustain, compared to many others fitness or sport goals around.

I have created The Wellness Sweet Spot to solve the paradox presented in the introduction of this book. Remember that, on one hand, we now have more free time "apparently," as all over the world, we have health and fitness clubs with incredible exercise machines, group classes, cheaper prices, and so on; we have many smart apps from companies like Nike Run Club; and the smartphones, watches, and wearables come with options to track physical activity and health. Furthermore, healthy food is all over nutritional stores. On the other hand, we have too much Physical Inactivity everywhere, with 80 percent of kids and more than 30 percent of adults, and these are conservative numbers.

Why is this spot sweet? Some of you may be wondering, "sweet?" It sounds high caloric or similar to diabetes, which is one of our worst enemies, but returning to the Tennis Sweet Spot analogy, remember that this spot is where the best shots in tennis are executed. It is the right place where the tennis ball should be hit with the racket's strings. It is so *sweet* when you hit it right. The ball gets more speed and power without extra effort when it goes out of the racket. The ball flies more accurately to the desired target in the opponent's court, and the sound when the ball is hit is *nice and sweet*. It is the same here—after some months of discipline, incorporating new healthy habits into our lives, doing our physical activity, watching our food intake, and doing some of the recommended quick tests like measuring our weight and waist, we will be feeling much better, happier, relaxed, alive, and so forth. And when our BMI is in the correct level, our waist-hip ratio is ok, our aerobic condition has improved considerably, and our physician has congratulated us because of the good results in our cholesterol test, we have hit the ball in the right place. *It is sweet to our hearth and soul, for we have reached The Wellness Sweet Spot.*

WHAT IS THE WELLNESS SWEET SPOT?

I think I got the answer to two of my questions with the formulation of the Wellness Sweet Spot; they are as follows:

WHAT REALLY MATTERS WHEN DOING SPORTS AND PHYSICAL ACTIVITY?

For me, after many years in this world of fitness and sports, *the answer is simple: Life.* What is more important, then? To win a World Cup or to abolish 100,000 deaths yearly by physical inactivity in a country? Or to win 50 Olympic gold medals in Tokyo 2020? Or to give a better, happier, and longer lives to 80,000,000 inhabitants? Or to pay an athlete $80,000,000 a year? Or to save 0.5 percent of the national GDP spent toward treating non-transmissible diseases (NCDs), which are easy to prevent by doing physical activity and taking a healthy diet? *So here we are talking about Life.*

HOW CAN WE FIND LIFE BY PRACTICING SPORTS AND PHYSICAL ACTIVITY?

By doing it wisely, I think, measuring our fundamental biometric elements in a friendly and easy manner and following the international health recommendations as those given by the WHO. I could say that The Wellness Sweet Spot synthetizes these recommendations and gives the pathway to higher levels of enjoyment and performance and *creates the bridge to bring those who are in the Life Risk Zones to a more safe and secure place.*

In one simple statement, **the Wellness Sweet Spot is Life!**

Let's keep analyzing the concept; in other words, the *Wellness Sweet Spot (WSS),* which is the physical condition level proposed in the Chapa Wellness Map model, where the risks of getting diseases related to physical inactivity have been diminished in an important manner through moderate and intense physical activity, sports, and a healthy diet.

Therefore, *I have created WSS looking for the most reliable level of physical condition for the majority of the world population.* I think it may be around 95 percent, because very few may want to, or can be able to, get to the High-Performance Level (I assume it could be 0.1% of the global population). Also, to get to the Fitness Level where the body looks almost perfect in shape and has all the physical-condition indicators in the correct levels (assuming 4.9% of the world population) requires many more resources, such as money, time, knowledge, effort, space, and so on; therefore, many people may have the desire to invest but not have the real interest in doing it, and many people all over the world just don't have those resources. However, unfortunately, we have the majority of the people in the planet below the *WSS*, living a Sedentary Lifestyle, so to teach them and encourage them to reach the *WSS* would be a good policy, public and private, because it is here where the health benefits come applying the optimal resources. *The Wellness Sweet Spot is a Zone of Optimization* so that much more people in the world could reach this spot, having successfully attained and sustained their more-educated and planned physical activity and sports goals.

Taking the meaning of Singularity as Extraordinary, we could say that The WSS is a Singularity Zone in the whole of today's sports and fitness industry, which we haven't had before, as presented in this book.

WHERE IS THE WELLNESS SWEET SPOT?

In the Chapa Wellness Map classification system, *the WSS is at the heart of this model*, and it is from where the solution for this Global Pandemic (Physical Inactivity) could be pumped. Graphically, in the model (see map in this chapter), it is right below the Fitness Level Zone and above the Active but not Enough Wellness Zone and promotes the use of Biometry Measurement Systems that the new technology is bringing to more people every day in a cheaper and friendly way all over the market. In the Chapa Wellness Map, the WSS is at the W7, W8, W9, and W10 levels, which are at the upper levels in the Green Wellness Circle at the center of this model; and for me is the Promise Land of Wellness (see map in this chapter).

You can find it very easily; just give the time and effort that your body deserves. What is the benefit of investing in health? What is the benefit of lowering the risk of diabetes or heart diseases? It is feeling your body alive, sweating more, and being slimmer, stronger, and stress-free, with an increased self-esteem. Here is where the Wellness Sweet Spot is; look for it!

We will be working hard during the forthcoming years to make the WSS worldwide known, to make it easy to find for almost everybody, to find ways where people can understand it better, find disruptive ways to apply it, and, above all, to help people to reach it out. Five million people are dying every year because of lack of understanding the importance of Physical Activity; billions of people in the planet—very sadly, many of them are kids—do not have the best present and possibly a worse future in terms of Well-Being.

WHAT ARE THE POSSIBLE APPLICATIONS?

I always try to see the practical applications of all these concepts so that in some chapters of this book, I have written some paragraphs in which I have given ideas of when and how it could be applied by some of the possible interested groups. In the previous chapter, I wrote about the potential uses of the Matrix 20 × 20, but I know I will write about the possibilities of the WSS.

People

Anyone could be helped to avoid frustration by focusing on more attainable and with more valuable objectives instead of striving to be like the good-looking model on the advertisement (that is not bad, but it does not work out for everybody). Also, people will be more encouraged about learning more about their bodies, biometry, nutrition, rest, training techniques, and so on. And they will get more of their smartphones' health applications, focusing on a very important issue: *to live longer and better.* The Wellness Sweet Spot could be used for all family members and could be a great motive for family integration. What a beautiful concept, don't you think so? *Unity through a Life promoting motive.*

Instructors and Trainers

Fitness instructors (Wellness instructors now), personal trainers, and coaches could use it to create programs that will be easier to understand, reach, and sustain, without getting their clients overtrained and burned out. Also, they may be able to create new exercises, techniques, and products for reaching this singular Sweet Spot. Also, by having their clients achieving their goals, in a systematic manner, they will be more successful with their clients and, therefore, in their careers. Club managers could develop marketing programs promoting the WSS full of benefits for anybody, and this zone will be easier to reach and sustain for many more club members, thereby *decreasing the attrition percentage* and helping the club to be more successful and profitable.

Universities

They could promote this Wellness Level for students and teachers who do not have much time because of their classes and assignments, but they could have the interest to reach this WSS by investing about five hours a week with a well-planned physical activity and/or sport. For students and teachers who are researchers in sciences related to this industry, like management, biology, medicine, chemistry, psychology, information technology, physical education, engineering, and so on, the WSS could give them an opportunity in this vast field of studies to develop knowledge for new technologies, products, systems, and so on, helping to achieve a global shift from Sedentarism to Physical Activism worldwide.

Hospitals

They could help to get the assessments to determine the Level of Wellness by Physical Activity of many people. Also, physicians could give medical programs to patients so that they could achieve and keep themselves in the WSS through exercise, a good nutritional regime, and on-time required health check-ups. Here would be a key change, with hospitals increasing their revenues in prevention with programs like Exercise is Medicine rather than in correction, which is wiser and cheaper, economically speaking, and allowing more free budget for patients, because they could use their savings for diseases not related to physical inactivity that would come sooner or later as they keep getting older.

NGOs

NGOs related to Health and Wellness could collaborate with the promotion of this WSS all over the world, partnering with the NGO World Wellness Network, so that physical activity programs would be adapted with food programs, motivating more kids and more people to *increase their lifespan and living standards* all over the world.

We have diet problems in many nations. The United Nations Food and Agriculture Organization (FAO) estimates that about 815,000,000 people (10.7%) in the world, out of the total 7,600,000,000, suffered from chronic undernourishment in 2016. This is alarming, but I also believe that in addition to food, we could find ways to take some Wellness by Physical Activity programs. Wherever and whenever would be possible; creativity and a good heart is necessary for this.

Economists

They may find in the WSS a more sustainable concept to elaborate economic policies, having in its core a cost benefit–oriented fundament where the *yields are not decreasing yet* as I believe we may be having in the Fitness and High-Performance levels. And this is a concept that could fit more in social programs because this is ego and vanity-free exercise for everybody, where economic savings will come by investing in a smarter, cost-effective manner.

Businessmen, Entrepreneurs, and CEOs

These could use this target to promote their Corporate Wellness programs in their offices and to attend the increasing requirements for healthier workplaces from governments as we can see it with the Luxembourg Declaration in the European Union, thus reaching the WSS by many workers. By this, a much productive and happier workplace will be accomplished. Many others would find in this industry an interesting investment opportunity due to the expected growing Wellness market for the forthcoming years.

Politicians

Politicians would find a more accurate and precise concept to promote better living for people in their political campaigns and could make their government plans more effective regarding health, well-being, social development, security, economy, children, demographic challenges, and sports programs. Can you imagine a complete district reaching the WSS that could be more historic than having a team winning seven world cups, something that any politician in the world could really present as a remarkable result?

But all starts at the personal level, when you have noticed how important it is to reach the Wellness Sweet Spot. Once you have known it, and when you have decided to go and get it, everything starts giving. . .

The first step, and I mean it literally.

CHAPTER 10

THE WORLD CLASSIFICATION SYSTEM FOR THE LEVELS OF WELLNESS THROUGH PHYSICAL ACTIVITY

Courage, my friends; 'tis not too late to build a better world.

—Tommy Douglas

CHAPA WELLNESS MAP

The aim of this chart is to present a statistical and trustworthy system of the classification of the levels of wellness by physical activity of the nations to compare a peridod of time with other and to have a world classification system where this variable will be considered as another important variable of the economic development of the nations.

WORLD MAP OF THE LEVELS OF WELLNESS BY PHYSICAL ACTIVITY

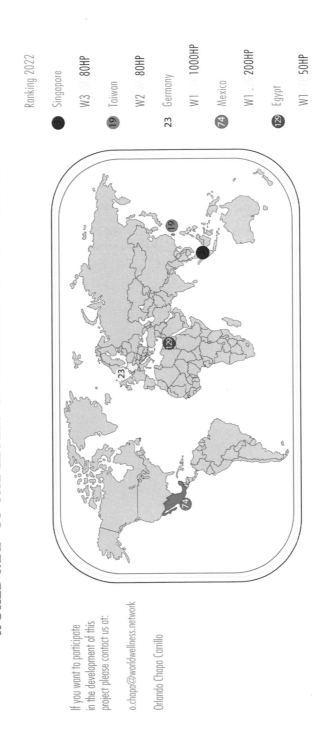

Ranking 2022

Singapore

W3 80HP

19 Taiwan

W2 80HP

23 Germany

W1 1000HP

74 Mexico

W1 200HP

129 Egypt

W1 50HP

If you want to participate
in the development of this
project please contact us at:

o.chapa@worldwellness.network

Orlando Chapa Carrillo

"These are just assumed values for this presentation that have to be changed after this project implementation."

Orlando Chapa

WHY DEVELOP A CLASSIFICATION SYSTEM FOR THE LEVELS OF WELLNESS THROUGH PHYSICAL ACTIVITY?

To End the Global Deaths Due to Physical Inactivity

Courage is needed to change something that has to be changed. In the previous chapter, we analyzed where we should be to have a more suitable place for good health—in other words, a Spot for Life. Courage is required, if we are not there, to move and to do something to get rid of the Risk Factors related to Physical Inactivity. The father of Canadian healthcare, Tommy Douglas, reminds us that we need courage to build a better world.

When I was writing the first lines of this chapter in May 2016, we were having a tough crisis all over the world, which was making many politicians of many countries think about going back to close borders, build walls, reduce international free trade, go back to be more nationalist, and stop globalization. This book is not about economics and geopolitics, but I believe that the world classification systems helps us to know more about us as nations by knowing more about other nations. I have seen and read many classification maps generated by the World Economic Forum, and I really think they are very helpful to improve the quality of life of the people to have a better world. Moreover, many of them are looking to attain the Sustainable Development Goals (SDGs) of the United Nations, which, in my personal view, is exciting.

So instead of learning by doing our own mistakes, we could cooperate between countries to learn from each other to, in this case, reduce the Global Mortality Rate due to Physical Inactivity, that it was calculated in 3,200,000 in the year 2012 by the World Health Organization and that, for today, some universities estimate that this number probably may be above 6,000,000.

To Better Politicians' Performance Measurements

I believe that in many countries, the way the Minister of Sports, Physical Culture, and other related activities presents the results of his administration sometimes falls short, because many times he or she is just focused on the amount of money invested in general infrastructure for sports and in the results that the national representative teams and athletes obtain in the competitions of a certain period of time or in a special event like the Olympic Games. By using this Classification System of the Levels of Wellness of Physical Activity, with a combination of a W for Wellness, with a number (from 1 to 10 according to each level of this segment in the Chapa Wellness Map); of an F for Fitness, with a number (a percentage); and with an HP for High-Performance, with a number starting from one to infinite (see map in this chapter), we could have a very complete report covering all the population of any country from a determined period of time, compared with another in the past, to see its improvement in the global rating from one year to another and from there search for the causes and look for solutions for the benefit of the governed people.

To Consider This Variable as an Important Measure of the Economic Development of the Nations

According to the SDGs (Sustainable Development Goals) of the ONU in Section 3 of a total of 17, the objective is to *ensure healthy lives and promote Well-Being for people of all ages* so that with this Classification System under the concepts of the Chapa Wellness Map model, we could propose that any developed nation as a modern developed nation should have a high level in this World Classification System, even though reaching a National Wellness Sweet Spot (NWSS) may be very hard to get (see map in chapter 11), even for the richest countries, because of the very bad habits that our Sedentary Society has today as a highly physically inactive culture. So beyond just watching the economic GDP growth and the increases in per capita income, the social Well-Being of the people of any nation could be considered to be part of a broader definition of development. Therefore, taking into consideration the Wellness Level of any nation, looking to end the deaths caused by physical inactivity, we will be counteracting the damages to our physical condition that the industrial revolutions have brought into our societies as a side effect. So developed nations must have a high rank in this classification system and developing nations must look to improve in this variable as a part of their goals, even though in some cases we may be able to find some developing nations with better Wellness using Physical Activity Ranking because of many cultural factors as Diet and Physical Activity at the workplace.

WHAT IS IT?

It is a system that will help us after its implementation to classify the countries all over the world to understand each population's the physical condition. It has three main segments to measure: Wellness (W), Fitness (F), and High-Performance (HP). Basically it helps us to be aware of where our priorities should go, where to invest, where to teach, where to direct public policy, and where to change, for the benefit of many. *This system is designed to be a tool for international cooperation above international competition;* higher rankings mean more people saved from death, and we will be looking to the best-ranked nations to learn from them what they are doing and share these practices and solutions to the rest of the world.

HOW IS IT CONSTITUTED?

I am placing as our main priority the Wellness (W) Level, which is where most of the population of each nation is; followed by the Fitness (F) Level, where not many people of any nation are; and finally to the High-Performance (HP) Level, where a very low percentage of the population belongs.

We are given with this a *Copernican Turn* in the design of the current model for the sports industry; *just as Earth is not at the center of the universe, High-Performance is not at the center of the industry now. Wellness is the shining star to look at, to where we direct our attention, and from where the Force of Gravity that makes the other elements move around comes.* This is a new paradigm shift, which will pay dividends to everybody.

For the Wellness, we should get the average of the whole population score, where we may be getting results in 2022—a national score of W3 for, let's say, Singapore. With this I am trying to say that the average of the physical condition of the population of Singapore is at the Level of Wellness 3. Let's assume that we did the same evaluation for Germany in the same year 2022 and that we got the result that the average of its population is in Wellness 1 (W1). These are just estimations used to illustrate the system.

As the second level of our new system, we could get the percentage of the people who are in the Fitness Level, as an example with estimated data; let's say, that in 2022, Singapore will have 0.5 percent of its population in the Fitness Level, and we will write it as 0.5 percent Fitness (0.5% F) and that Germany will have a score of 0.2 percent Fitness (0.2% F).

Finally, we will get the score of these two nations at the High-Performance Level. Keeping with the same example, let's think that after the evaluation we have gotten that in 2022, Singapore has 80 points for High-Performance, expressed as 80 High-Performance (80 HP), and that Germany for the same year has gotten 1,000 points, 1,000 High-Performance (1,000 HP). I am using a points systems for the High-Performance Level, where all the International Sports Events and Competitions will give points to each country for the classification system, depending on the result and the difficulty of the competition; for example, a *bronze medal* in the Olympic games will give more HP points than a Gold medal in a European Tournament, or being finalist in the Soccer World Cup will give more HP points than winning the Copa America in Soccer.

Continuing with this scenario, we have the 2022 Classification for two countries:

Singapore: W3 0.5F 80HP

Germany: W1 0.2F 1000HP

Here I would like to present another important point of this system that I am creating, and it is to give a higher priority in the Classification System to the Wellness Level; therefore, the countries will focus their Sports and Physical Activity Public Policy to improve their Wellness Level, at their lower levels, where most of the people are and where almost all the health problems related to Physical inactivity come from. Therefore, keeping with the same example, we may get the following classification for these two countries, already having evaluated many countries:

Singapore: W3 0.5F 80HP, World Rank # 3

Germany: W1 0.2F 1000HP, World Rank # 23

We can notice in this assumed scenario that even though Germany has 12.5 times more points in the High-Performance Level—a very powerful athletic nation in the Olympic Games and Football Soccer Cups—Singapore is ranked higher, number 3 in the world, because it has a higher level of Wellness and because it has a national population average of W3, which, even though is still low and far of the National Wellness Sweet Spot, has a more physically active population than Germany (this is just for an example). I believe that if we can make this system Mathematically Precise, that is my desire, and this book is also an invitation to make that happen. We could help to reduce the Global Pandemic of Physical Inactivity in an important manner; it is focused to give priority to improve the Wellness Level of the nations, understanding Wellness as it is defined in this book.

Another important point is that I am giving more priority to the people at the Fitness Level than to the people at the High-Performance Level. By this I am saying that in case we may be having two countries with the same evaluation in Wellness and with different High-Performance points and different percentage of people in Fitness, we will be given a better position in the ranking system to the nation that has the higher percentage of Fitness. Fitness has a higher priority in this classification system, although the nation ranked lower because of their lower percentage of population in Fitness could have had more High-Performance points. In other words, a nation with an evaluation of W3 0.5F 100HP will have a higher global classification than a nation with an evaluation of W3 0.2F 500HP.

W>F>HP: Wellness > Fitness > High-Performance

HOW IS IT TO BE DONE AND IMPLEMENTED?

After publishing this book in 2019, we will be ready to create the system. Then, through the NGO World Wellness Network, which will be founded soon, the system will be implemented so as to start getting the first countries evaluations and classifications, and we will begin to support them to improve their scores and ranking in practical ways. We will need the collaboration of many, from all over the world, and with many backgrounds to make this task happen.

WHEN?

This book will be in print in 2019 and the system ready by 2021; therefore, I believe we could start getting the first national evaluations in 2022.

WHERE?

All over the world, we have made contact with some nations such as Germany, the United States, Slovenia, Austria, Mexico, Holland, Turkey, Spain, among other countries. And all the people who were asked, want to participate. We are in the early stages of the project, and I believe that as soon as the project starts to grow, many more nations would like to be part of it.

Just remember that the most important part of this whole system is you!
Your life matters to us.

So let's keep working!

CHAPTER 11

GLOBAL W7

*To accomplish great things, we must not only act but
also dream, not only plan but also believe.*

—Anatole France

GLOBAL W7

CHAPA WELLNESS MAP

On this chart I am presenting two scenarios, both assumed. The initial one where I think that is where the world is currently today, as if THE CLASSIFICATION SYSTEM OF THE LEVELS OF WELLNESS BY PHYSICAL ACTIVITY has been already applied; and the final scenario, where I think that is where the world could be by the year 2030; assuming the application of the same system to evaluate the world, and that all the concepts of the CHAPA WELLNESS MAP and more have been already implemented in many nations.

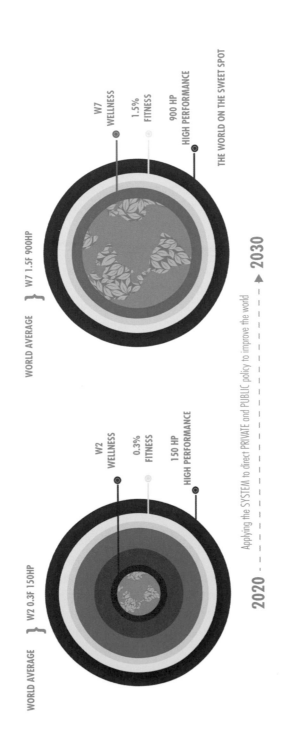

WORLD AVERAGE } W2 0.3F 150HP

W2
WELLNESS

0.3%
FITNESS

150 HP
HIGH PERFORMANCE

WORLD AVERAGE } W7 1.5F 900HP

W7
WELLNESS

1.5%
FITNESS

900 HP
HIGH PERFORMANCE

THE WORLD ON THE SWEET SPOT

2020 - - - - - - - - - - - Applying the SYSTEM to direct PRIVATE and PUBLIC policy to improve the world - - - - - - - - - ▸ 2030

*a) On this scenario we have the world population in an average of WELLNESS LEVEL 2, with .3% of the global population in FITNESS LEVEL and each country having an average of 150 points in HIGH PERFORMANCE LEVEL.

**b) On this second scenario, an ideal one for the world we could say, we have the world population in an average of WELLNESS LEVEL 7, with 1.5% of the global population in FITNESS LEVEL and each country having an average of 900 points in HIGH PERFORMANCE LEVEL.

Orlando Chapa

127

LET'S DREAM A LITTLE

In chapter 6, I quoted, *"There are things known and there are things unknown, and in-between are the doors of perception.,"* from the author Aldous Huxley, and now that I will be writing about a dream for a better world, his book came to my mind—*Brave New World*—where Huxley himself refers to his book as a negative utopia or dystopia, because in 1931, when this novel was written, he anticipated developments in reproductive technology, sleep-learning, psychological manipulation, among other technologies, that would have brought important changes in society at that time, which, in many ways, could have brought negative effects to the society in those days.

To increase the Levels of Wellness by Physical Activity, to get a Global Classification of Wellness 7 (W7) or above as the world average, according to the Chapa Wellness Map, I believe this could be almost a utopia. But I also believe it could be a reachable goal with all the smart technology and connectivity that this Fourth Industrial Revolution is bringing to more people day by day all over the world, with the population awareness of the need to become physically more active in many countries and increasing day by day all over, with the help of NGOs as the World Wellness Network and many others helping the nations to develop public policies toward getting people more physically active, with sports businesses targeting the Wellness segment with new innovative products and services, with mothers and fathers teaching their kids to do exercise and to eat better, with innovative ideas in media and social media to promote Wellness, and so on.

But how bad a Global W7 could be? I answer to that saying: not bad at all. To express it in simpler words, a Global W7 is having the majority of the population of the world doing five hours or more a week of planned physical activity and eating in a healthy way; that is all! So I believe that this goal would be a positive "utopia." Or, instead of that, to have a Global W7, it would be a feasible global goal. What do you think?

According to chapter 3, the ONU has established as SDGs for 2030 to ensure healthy lives and promote Well-Being for all at all ages; reduce maternal mortality ratio; end preventable deaths of newborns and children under five years of age; end the epidemics of AIDS, tuberculosis, and malaria; and reduce hepatitis, among other important goals. What do you think about including the Global W7 goal for 2030? We may end with the deaths related to not being in this healthy Wellness Sweet Spot that causes between 3,300,000 and more than 6,000,000 deaths every year all over the world. Physical Inactivity is a serious enemy and has to be defeated soon!

Let's think a little bit in other scenarios just to exercise the mind. How would a global High-Performance 1 (HP1) be? Is this is really a utopia? Is almost everybody in the world an athlete? Are all of us an amateur or, in a higher HP level, a professional player? This is impossible to achieve and not even a good goal that all the people may like, so let's dismiss it. Therefore, High-Performance from HP1 to HP5 is a feasible aspirational goal for very few in the planet.

And what about a global F1 (Fitness 1)? I cannot imagine almost everybody in perfect shape, looking fit, with biometry and biochemistry (cholesterol and triglycerides) tests in correct levels, doing more than 10 hours a week of planned moderate or intense physical activity, having good levels in all the skill factors of fitness like speed and strength, and keeping an almost perfect diet. This would be a nice dream probably for Arnold Schwarzenegger or Sylvester Stallone or my father, Zovek. But I believe that this is almost impossible to achieve, at least in this century, if someday this would be a desirable goal for everybody. Therefore, Fitness from F1 to F5 in the Chapa Wellness Map is a feasible aspirational goal for some.

A Global W1 (Wellness 1) means that the average global physical condition of the whole world is in the Sedentary Zone. We are moving in the right direction as many of the world's population is getting into Physical Activity, Fitness, and High-Performance and that they are increasing the global average above a total W1 score. Therefore, a Global Wellness 1 (W1), and all the way through Wellness 3 (W3) in our Map, where almost all the problems of physical inactivity come from, is not a desirable goal but a side effect of our modern society. I say this because my forecast for the Global Wellness Level measured today is of a W2 (see map in this chapter).

Having a Global W4 (Wellness 4) could be not too bad a score for the whole world, because this would mean that the average of the global population is describing that the people are getting physically more active and eating healthier, doing it *Better but not Enough*. The people in general would be getting away from that Sedentary Lifestyle that is killing us; this could be an incredible trend, but people in this case would be keeping the risk of contracting diseases caused due to being physically inactive; that is our main goal and the *Key Factor that describes the Wellness Sweet Spot*. This level could be a good medium-term goal for a global score.

Therefore, *a Global W7 (Wellness 7)—a Global Wellness Sweet Spot*, where we can find from W7 through W10 levels, W7 being the first level of this Sweet Spot possible to reach, where we can already find all the benefits described in chapter 9—*is the best, more convenient, and feasible optional level to have as a Global Classification*, obviously after heavy hard work from many to get it implemented in all global levels and the enough physical activity and discipline of the world's population. This scenario is where we could have *zero deaths* attributed to Physical Inactivity.

Now, let's keep analyzing some scenarios to grasp more understanding of this Model.

How Would the World Look With a Score of W2 0.3F 150HP?

This may be as I see it, the current state of the world, in this Classification System, where the average of all the population would be W2 (Wellness 2), as I have noticed in many nations that I have visited, such as Israel, Jordan, Greece, Italy, Vatican City State, Slovenia, Austria, Czech Republic, Switzerland, Germany, France, Spain, Belgium, Holland, Finland, England, Ireland, the United States, Japan, Taiwan, and Mexico. And because of all the national and global reports that I have studied related to Physical Inactivity, which are resumed in the First Chapter of this book, very few people do physical activity and exercise in a planned and continuous way, keeping a healthy diet. 0.3F (0.3 Fitness), where I am estimating that this is the state today, where just about 0.3 percent of the world population is in the Fitness LEVEL, as described in Chapter 8, and that each nation has an average of 150HP (150 High-Performance points), meaning that after all the international competitions, including the points given from all the professional leagues in each country, the whole world's High-Performance points given divided by all the countries evaluated, results in 150HP points per nation (this is an estimated number as if this Classification System would have been finished and applied, just to exemplify the use of the Chapa Wellness Map).

As you may have noticed, the most relevant evaluation here is the W2; this means that as an average, the world population is doing about two or three hours per week of Physical Activity, that we have Overweight and Obesity in an important manner all over, that the Waist-Hip ratio is not accurate for many, and that in general we are getting bad results in all the biometry tests considered in the Matrix 20 × 20 mentioned in chapter 8. And the relevant point here is that this is the reason why we are having from 3.3 to more than 6 million deaths worldwide every year.

I really think that the Wellness State of the World today is close to this assumed result, and for me this is so sad, because of the costs and discomfort it generates and also because I really believe it wouldn't be very complicated to start to reverse it.

What If the Whole World Had a Score of W7 1.5F 900HP by 2030?

This would be great. This is the world having a Global W7, as we discussed a little at the beginning of this chapter, but now I am going to explain deeper how growing from a W2 to a W7 would influence a growth in F (Fitness) and HP (High-Performance) levels as well. I believe that with more than 30 percent of adults and 80 percent of kids not doing the enough recommended Physical Activity, moving to the W7 Level, this will generate more people reaching the Fitness Level, and this has to be revised statistically; but I think that the world could move from a 0.3F (0.3 Fitness) to as far as a 1.5F (1.5 Fitness). Why do I believe this could happen? Because many more people getting closer to the Fitness Circle will be motivated to have the Shape of a Fit Body and, being already in the Sweet Spot, approximately just half of the way to be 100 percent FIT. For those who have the resources, motivation, and will to go for the Yellow Fitness Level, I believe they will get it. We have a growing club industry that could handle this very well. The High-Performance Zone could also benefit greatly, because people, families, schools, workplaces, public places, and more getting Physicalle Active will motivate more kids and teenagers to give their hearts and lives full time to their favorite sport. With more of them getting involved and with the disruptive expansion of the industry, obviously new sports and more competitions at the High-Performance Level will be generated; therefore, more points coming out from more international events would come, resulting in an increase in the High-Performance points of each nation, generating a higher global average that I think could reach 900HP in 2030 compared to 150HP in 2020, which I assume as the condition in the year 2020 (see map in this chapter).

How Could This Be Done?

In the introduction of this book, I talked about a world Wellness chain reaction that brings and sustains life. I believe that if 1 percent of the world population may be able to get their level of Wellness through Physical Activity in the year 2022, we could get each nation's ranking with statistical methods, and through the NGO World Wellness Network interacting with many other NGOs, we could help each interested country to reach more people to know their level and to move up to a higher level and to a healthier lifestyle. Another Key Factor, I believe, will come from the current clubs, gyms, sports centers, hospitals, schools, universities, workplaces, government offices, Internet, apps, and so on, to start to get their members classification and, with the use of modern technology as Apps and Social Networks, spread the project and the assessments everywhere.

Definitively the support and involvement of governments, with the financial help of private companies and media, a win-win-win virtuous circle could happen to know each nation's score and rating with the intention to improve it. This would make the Global W7 a goal that could be attainable in the near future. But if organizations like the OMS, ONU, World Economic Forum, and so on, could recognize this goal as one of SDGs, I think this could happen by the year 2030. I have to point out that while I was writing this book, I invited many universities and researchers from all over the world to this project, and the response has been very positive; I can just feel gratitude for their interest in improving these approaches and ideas to a level of international approval.

What Is the Cost of a Global W7?

We have 3,300,000 to more than 6,000,000 deaths and increasing every year due to Physical Inactivity. I wonder how much we could spend to save one person of those millions. We are now passing through a very tough global economic crisis, which sometimes looks as a dead-end street, so that governments are having a shoestring budget; individuals and families are also tied in their spending. The same is the case with many corporations. But if we have a 1.1 percent of the global GDP applied to the whole sports industry, I believe we can do better with *innovation* and *new approaches* focusing on finishing this Global Pandemic, having do-it-yourself physical activity programs for people of all ages, activating ourselves while watching sports on TV, taking 10-minute workout break at work every two hours, and so on. These actions will not cost too much using free Internet channels, such as YouTube or Facebook. These are just examples of the possible initiatives that could be done in the very short term, as we have seen others during the exposition of this book.

Let's remember that governments are spending an important part of the health budget correcting instead of preventing all the diseases related to Physical Inactivity. If we would start applying part of that budget to help create this local, then national, and finally global chain reaction, governments will soon have savings in the health budgets and apply part of those savings to diseases unrelated to physical inactivity, thereby increasing in this manner each nation's life-span. So any possible present cost "investment" will become a great gain in the medium and long term.

Here we are not taking in consideration the private initiative, where I think many current sport, fitness, wellness, health, technological, and so on, companies and many new start-ups could act in a very proactive way, using all the technological transformation that we are starting to live today to grow this market, improving the score of each person, and thus the nationals and the global results, making good business out of these enterprises and, above all, *saving lives!*

Slovenia, an Example of Good Practices

In April 2016 and 2017, I was invited to two symposiums in Ljubljana, Slovenia, in the subject of Healthy Lifestyle, one each year, where more than 20 speakers from all over the world talked about very interesting topics for the health promotion for all ages and in the workplaces. Besides getting to know many friendly PhDs from more than six nations, I got impressed about how a small population country like Slovenia, whose population is around 2,000,000 people, compared with let's say Mexico, which has around 120,000,000 people, has so much interest in improving the health of its population through exercise and healthy habits programs, such as bike riding all over the cities, healthier workplaces, health and fitness centers, smart apps, and with the continuous presentation of congresses and symposia, looking among other goals to achieve the recommendations of the Luxembourg Declaration in Workplace Health Promotion.

This declaration for the European Union nations believes that "a healthy, motivated, and well-qualified workforce is fundamental to the future social and economic well-being of the European Union." They also believe that the concept of Workplace Health Promotion (WHP) "is the combined efforts of employers, employees, and society to improve the health and well-being of people at work."

"Healthy people in healthy organizations" is an awesome statement of this declaration, which I really think should be followed by all the countries of the world; Chapa Map model "fits" perfectly for these types of initiatives.

So I just can't stop sharing this example with whosoever may have interest in wherever I go; it is inspiring.

Well done, Slovenia!

PART III

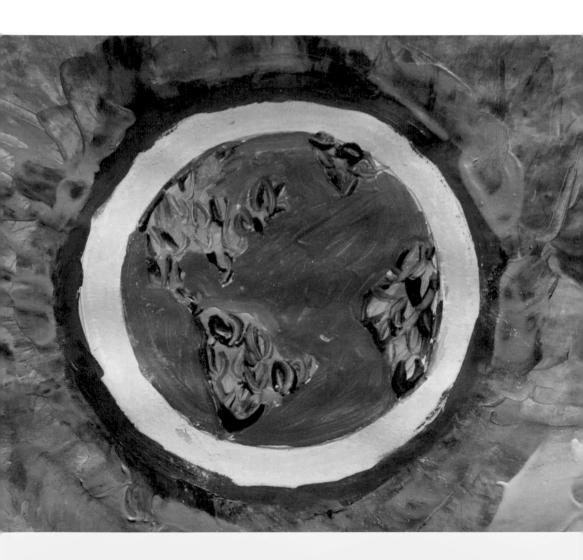

CHAPTER 12

AUF GEHTS!: WORLD WELLNESS NETWORK

Give me a place to stand, and I will move the earth.

—Archimedes

AUF GEHT S

WORLD WELLNESS NETWORK

CHAPA WELLNESS MAP

ALL STARTS WITH YOU

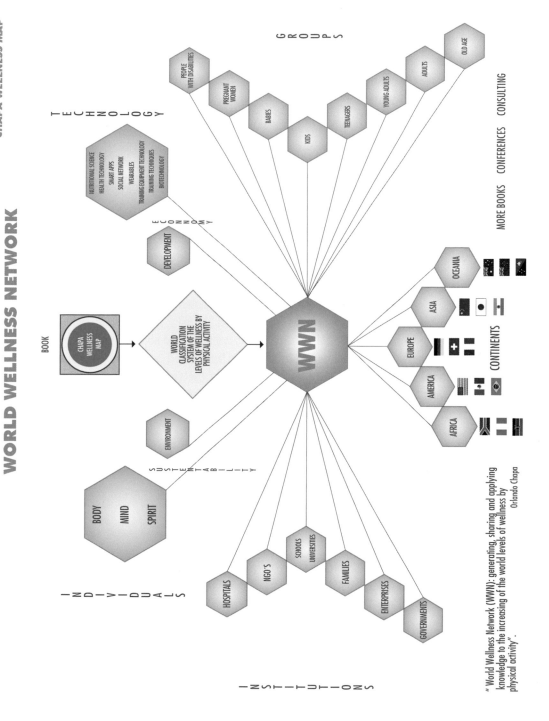

BOOK

CHAPA WELLNESS MAP

WORLD CLASSIFICATION SYSTEM OF THE LEVELS OF WELLNESS BY PHYSICAL ACTIVITY

WWN

T E C H N O L O G Y

NUTRITIONAL SCIENCE
HEALTH TECHNOLOGY
SMART APPS
SOCIAL NETWORK
WEARABLES
TRAINING EQUIPMENT TECHNOLOGY
TRAINING TECHNIQUES
BIOTECHNOLOGY

E C O N O M Y

DEVELOPMENT

ENVIRONMENT

S U S T E N T A B I L I T Y

BODY
MIND
SPIRIT

I N D I V I D U A L S

G R O U P S

PEOPLE WITH DISABILITIES
PREGNANT WOMEN
BABIES
KIDS
TEENAGERS
YOUNG ADULTS
ADULTS
OLD AGE

CONTINENTS

OCEANIA
ASIA
EUROPE
AMERICA
AFRICA

MORE BOOKS   CONFERENCES   CONSULTING

HOSPITALS
NGO'S
SCHOOLS
UNIVERSITIES
FAMILIES
ENTERPRISES
GOVERNMENTS

I N S T I T U T I O N S

" World Wellness Network (WWN): generating, sharing and applying knowledge to the increasing of the world levels of wellness by physical activity". -
Orlando Chapa

137

A SURPRISE

In New Year's season at the end of 2015, I was spending some time with family in Aachen, Germany, after attending some trade shows in Barcelona and Germany, contacting some universities at Spain, Germany, and Switzerland and visiting some NGOs in Geneva. A great surprise came to me in about a two-week period. It happened that one evening a friend and his wife from the district of Richterich, Aachen, Germany, knew that I was writing this book, the *Chapa Wellness Map*; they were so interested about my idea of creating a map to have a global picture of the world population's physical condition, because of the Costs of Physical Inactivity, that I shared with them the whole project, and they were very kind in listening to me, showing a genuine interest for it, for which I will always be grateful to them because that encouraged me so much to keep writing this book with a global vision.

But that was not all! The next two weeks in Aachen, in some districts close to Richterich, I saw all kind of people of all ages doing Physical Activity all over the places. I saw seniors jogging, kids roller-skating and riding bikes, fathers with their babies in tandem bikes, people running with their dogs or hiking on the hills, many people walking with their family members, some others doing Nordic walking, and so on. There were so many and in so many places that I could say that if it had lasted at least six months, we for sure could have had the first district in the world in the Wellness 7 level (the first level in the Sweet Spot). But, unfortunately, that Wellness "carnival" just lasted the holidays; nevertheless, it was very impressive and inspirational to me. Thank you, Aachen, and thanks to the people, friends, and family of Richterich and of the other districts for that gift; just by being there and watching that was a great gift. *Vielen Dank! (Thank you very much! - ¡Muchas gracias!)*

THE BOOK

So auf gehts! translated from German to English is *here we go!* Thus, the first stage of this project was writing this book, the *Chapa Wellness Map*, where we have been presenting the general idea and the basic concepts of A Systematic Approach to Physical Activity, where I have established the following:

a) Three main zones: Wellness, Fitness, and High Performance.

b) That we should look for a more feasible, easier-to-reach-and-to-sustain zone as a goal for people's physical activity level, The Wellness Sweet Spot (from W7 to W10), in the Chapa Wellness Map Classification System.

c)   That it would be very useful to have a World Classification System of the Levels of Wellness by Physical Activity.

d)   That the foundation of the NGO World Wellness Network will be key for the global implementation of this project in the coming years.

e)   And finally that the most important part in all this is you. Dear reader, if you are not doing the recommended Physical Activity, start to move right now, and do something to change that inactive lifestyle. My advice is that if you are not doing five hours per week of physical activity, stop reading, and if you don't have any prohibition of your doctor, go and walk for at least 30 minutes and come back to keep reading.

I am very happy while writing this particular chapter, the last chapter of this first book, although I will be writing some other very interesting themes for the Special Topics and Epilogue sections, like how we can obtain our current level of Wellness by Physical Activity and the application of this model in a bank or in a city (getting the title of Wellness City) because of their infrastructure and programs, and so on. I am very happy because I have been applying myself the concepts presented here, doing my daily jogging, walking, strength routine, eating less calories, and so on, and very soon I will be back on the WSS. I am also sharing some of the findings of my research and insights with my family, friends, and neighbors, and they are listening. You know, sometimes it is hard to get with people and tell them that the WHO recommends to have a BMI less than 24.9 or a Waist-to-Hip ratio below .90 in men and .85 in women; it is so hard to tell people about these sensitive topics that nobody really speaks about this when you are not in the gym or club. I mean we must be slimmer, which is not fashion; in other words, many, many people all over are overweight or worst. The recommendations of the highest health authorities in the world suggest that we must eat less and move more. But, you know, because of the people that I know are listening, I am very happy I haven't been punched yet! And some of them are increasing their Physical Activity and listening that they have to check some corporal measurements to be in a less-risky health situation.

So this book is undergoing a transformation, like myself, *from a Systematic Approach to Physical Activity to Be Active, Be Well, Be Alive.* And that makes me really happy, because the center of this model, a new model for the Sports Industry, is you, not the millionaire athlete who is all over the media, not the incredible-looking magazine model showing her almost perfect body symmetry, not the owner of a big sporting goods company or a fitness center. The center of our efforts is you—you who weren't aware of the need to *move more* up to a *safer spot* for a longer and better life to, let's say, a spot that could make the last 30 years of your life the best ones ever, combining a healthy body with a mature mind.

That's what I want for you!

THE CLASSIFICATION SYSTEM

Thus, the first stage of this project is *you, starting to move into the Wellness Sweet Spot,* and that means giving the first step, as my father Zovek once wrote, "The journey of the 1,000 kilometers starts with the first step." If you want, you can know your level in the Chapa Wellness Map right now. Just go to the letter a) in the next section of this book; it will take you just a few minutes, and you can come back to keep reading this chapter that presents the general idea of this exciting world project.

Now we can go further to the second stage, that is, to get the Level of Wellness by Physical Activity of the 1 percent of the people of one section of a city. With this, we can get to know the approximate score of a complete section. Knowing this number, we can look for the results of another section in the same city, using the same method. We have the Internet, schools, universities, companies, hospitals, smart apps, and so on, to reach people. Knowing the Wellness Level of some districts or sections of a city, we can calculate the score of that particular city; this could help us to get the Wellness Levels of the interested people in many cities and towns. Soon we could have enough data to calculate the score of a state of an interested nation; once we have all the states of a country, we will be in a position to have the first Level of Wellness by Physical Activity of a nation. With this I think we will be ready to get to know the score of other countries with the NGO that will be formed—World Wellness Network (WWN).

THE NGO "WORLD WELLNESS NETWORK"

This NGO that will be formed, the third stage, will implement the project to have the Classification System of the Levels of Wellness by Physical Activity all over the World, and this NGO will help all the countries that want to receive support to improve in their ranking, through the *generation, sharing, and the application of knowledge related to the increasing of healthier lifestyles in the population, which will reduce the levels of mortality associated with Physical Inactivity.*

The first task here will be to generate the World Wellness by Physical Activity Ranking, at least of the first 10 countries involved for the year 2022; from there, go for more and more nations to classify in the Chapa Wellness Map. The next step will be to create a team that will work full time in the NGOs' headquarters in Germany, and national representatives will be developed in each country to work together with many universities, NGOs, governments, institutes, research centers, companies, hospitals, individuals, and so on, to develop solutions, ideas, technology, and public policy *to share good practices* with all the nations involved with the goal of increasing the ranking of each nation, resulting in the improvement of the global average, *looking to the Global Wellness Sweet Spot* by the year 2030. Aggressive objective, don't you think? But many people are dying today, and we most move forward right now.

The NGO World Wellness Network (WWN) will be inclusive in many ways, having in mind the searching and development of solutions to improve the physical condition of people with disabilities, pregnant women, babies, kids, teenagers, young adults, adults, elders, ethnic groups, prisons, and so on, teaching them about the Wellness Sweet Spot and helping them to reach that goal. The WWN will be connected with institutions like families, schools, universities, hospitals, companies, governments, and NGOs, supporting them and being supported by them in all possible ways, looking for the increasing of the Levels of Wellness by Physical Activity of the people who want to do it and educating them of the need to have a healthier lifestyle of those who don't want to.

Our vision goes to every continent where we know that different challenges will be faced. Africa, as we know, is facing poverty with low economic growth. Here it may sound luxurious to do exercise, but we know that everybody needs to do it in a balanced way, so we must find ways to give the basic concepts of Wellness while helping them to end hunger. Obesity is prevalent in the United States and Mexico, and Latin America needs economic growth to be inclusive so that inequality would be reduced, so to integrate Physical Activity in people's lifestyle could be a good goal here. Asia has been driving the world economic growth, but inequality and poverty remains; two-thirds of the world's poor live here. Therefore, programs of public and social physical Wellness could be proposed here. Europe now faces the Brexit, the Greek crisis, the refugee crisis, the threat of terrorism, and extreme nationalism, but I really believe that the aging of its population and the costs of diabetes and heart disease could be added here as important challenges to overcome; therefore, with the option of applying Wellness programs for better aging, lowering medical expenses, and reducing the costs caused by overweight and obesity could be good goals in Europe, with the increase in Physical Activity in children and adolescents, where also we have a problem. Finally, there is Oceania, where poverty in rural areas is present besides all the problems that modernity has brought to the cities; thus, innovation to develop low cost physical Wellness programs are required here. So more precise studies and solutions are necessary all over; we have too much work to do ahead of us, in a world that needs to keep working together in better ways to solve many global challenges.

MORE BOOKS, CONFERENCES, CONSULTING

I am very happy that people in different places have asked me for conferences, to write more books, and for consulting. I feel very excited when I think that this book could be in the hands of many people all over the world, helping to change lives for good, helping to change paradigms for good, and helping to change industries for good. We are talking about many lives that could be saved by just moving more, activating, doing exercise, doing some easy healthy check-ups, learning how to eat the right quantity and quality of food, and learning to enjoy doing it. Because we have living bodies that need oxygen and nutrients, with muscles and bones that have to be strengthened, just like our heart, it is just a matter of changing habits.

The next book that will be written in these series Chapa Wellness Map will be one that is going to be focused in the Workplace. In the second chapter of this first book, we saw the historic evolution of the intensity of Physical Activity related to the way we work, and we have analyzed very briefly that one of the most important spaces where this Global Pandemic started is at the Workplace; therefore, we must correct it there, and we have seen many of the costs to corporations that this problem has brought in the form of absenteeism, presenteeism, and lack of productivity.

The third book that I will write will focus in the private sector, in business, looking to capitalize many opportunities that the Technological Revolution that this Industry 4.0 is giving us, of course applying the Chapa Wellness Map strategic management tool. I will present 100 new disruptive Wellness ideas of business that doesn't exist, all of them looking to *accomplish the goal of bringing to zero the global deaths due to physical inactivity;* in other words, taking the Planet to a level of W7 or more as a global average. It will be a strong call for entrepreneurs and start-up developers; this is my vision for the third writing adventure.

Conferences? I think that universities, corporations, government, and global institutions to get to know and apply the Wellness Sweet Spot it will be necessary; and to promote a change in the Current Sports Model, some conferences will have to be given in the current fitness industry trade shows to reach gyms, clubs, fitness centers, equipment manufacturers, service providers, and so on, and also in the sporting goods industry to make a call to solve this Global Pandemic with disruptive approaches in business. This also includes many other forums with entrepreneurs and business management students to invite them to invest in this redefined Wellness industry, which has a highly prominent future and which has been challenged today for this unsolved Physical Inactivity Pandemic. This will be a good field to sow these Wellness concepts.

The private sector will require consulting to help their employees to reach the Wellness Sweet Spot and more; and the Wellness, Fitness, and Sports industry companies might require support, to gain good market participation during the significant Wellness industry growth that will come, that, as we have commented, could be tripled in the next 12 years.

WORLD WELLNESS CHAIN REACTION STARTS WITH YOU!

Everything starts with you. You have to give the first step in this war against Physical Inactivity. This is your foe, in letter a), in the next section "Special Topics," where, in very few minutes, you can know your level of Wellness by Physical Activity. Just to know the size of our enemy, let's take a look at this information: in 2016, the top 10 causes of death around the world according to the World Health Organization were:

1. Ischemic heart disease

2. Stroke

3. Chronic obstructive pulmonary disease

4. Lower respiratory infections

5. Alzheimer disease

6. Trachea, bronchus, lung cancers

7. Diabetes mellitus

8. Road injury

9. Diarrheal diseases

10. Tuberculosis

Physical Inactivity encompasses 6 percent of them, with more than 3.3 million (the World Economic Forum has published that there are more than 5 million), being the fourth cause of death. So now that you know your enemy, my hope is that you start to attack it as soon as possible. You just have to move, consult your physician, and enjoy a change of life; and if you are already doing your recommended Physical Activity or more, my desire is that the Chapa Wellness Map model, books, and classification system can help you to keep doing and to keep growing your personal Wellness for many years.

THE **CHAPA WELLNESS MAP**

I have calculated that if you can tell two family members or friends or peers at work, if each one of us can make aware two other persons of *the need to move, to be physically active*, to look for the correct levels of BMI and Waist-Hip Ratio to start, and if this happens on and on, in less than 33 times, I mean, 33 times one person tells another two persons, and each one of these two persons tells another two persons, and so on, we will be reaching all the population of the world:

$2^{32.8} = 7{,}477{,}972{,}397.74$ people

This is just a mathematical exercise to show some numbers, in a method that probably in the real world may have many hindrances and won't work, but I just want to show that it wouldn't be so hard and expensive if we really understand that we can save more than 5,000,000 lives every year if we can understand this situation and share this possible solution, with a sincere heart, that *we need to move*. With the discipline to do our daily Physical Activity to change our Sedentary Lifestyle, we can start defeating this subtle enemy.

In Article 25 (1) of the Universal Declaration of Human Rights proclaimed in the United Nations General Assembly in Paris on December 10, 1948, it was established that—

"Everyone has the right to a standard of living adequate for the health and well-being of himself and of his family . . ."

As Archimedes has said, let's move the earth.
Auf gehts!

PART IV

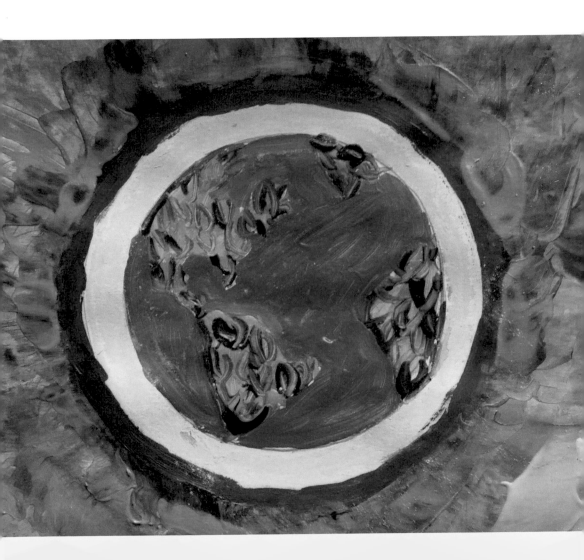

SPECIAL TOPICS

In this section, I will be talking briefly of some subjects that are very important for physical Wellness, but I intentionally have not included them in the Chapa Wellness Map chapters so as not to make them too complicated but only those that are necessary, since *a Healthy Lifestyle requires a holistic approach.* Also now, any person will be able to know now his or her initial Wellness Level to start to look for a better one, or remain in the same, in the case it is a convenient one.

FIND OUT YOUR WELLNESS LEVEL NOW!

Ok, let's start to evaluate in an easy and practical way our physical condition according to the Chapa Wellness Map classification system. Just by answering a very few questions, you will have your *Initial Level*, which will be very helpful to localize where you are and where you should be or to where you may want to go. To confirm your Wellness Level, it will require many tests that are not really necessary right now, but once you start to get more committed with your Wellness program, you will need to do them to get your level in a more precise way. This one that you are going to get now is more practical because the lower Levels of Wellness are not very hard to overcome. *If you really want to live better, you just have to move more and eat in an intelligent and measured manner* so that by the time you would like to get more evaluations, for sure you will be in a higher level in the Chapa Wellness Map. On the other hand, if you are in the higher levels, the most probable is that you are already deep involved in these kinds of tests, and they are being done by very competent specialists.

We will start with the questions for the higher levels—High-Performance and Fitness—and when we get into the Wellness queries, we will move from the lower levels of Wellness up to the Wellness Sweet Spot. For now this system will apply for adults from 18 to 64 years old; soon I will create the Chapa Wellness Map Classification System for Kids and Adolescents too, from 5 to 17 years old; by the way Diego, Irina's son (Irina is my niece), when he was just nine years old, made a weekly physical activity program for kids when I was starting to write this book in Aachen, which he must begin to apply soon because he has been gaining some weight lately. And a Classification System specialized for seniors, older than 65 years old, is required as well.

Notes: *To obtain your BMI, you must divide your weight in kilograms by the square of your height in meters (weight kg / (height meters × height meters)).

**To obtain your Waist-Hip Ratio, you must measure your waist and divide it by your hip. Just make sure to use the same scale, centimeters, meters, inches, and so on, because it is a Ratio (waist cm / hip cm or waist inches / hip inches, etc.). The most practical method recommended to measure your waist circumference (size) is to do it at the point of the minimal size; for the hip circumference (size), do it at the widest portion of the buttocks. The tape while you measure your waist circumference (size) and your hip circumference (size) must be tight to the skin of your body but not too much, and you must use a measuring tape that doesn't stretch when you pull it, changing the size of the metric scale.

***If your work (labor) demands heavy or moderate physical activity, such as construction, agriculture, lifting objects, too much walking, and so on, it is probable that your level may be higher. In such cases, the determinant factors to know your final level will be your BMI, Waist-Hip Ratio, Aerobic Condition, Blood Chemistry, and the other assessments. *The hours of physical activity are very important, but what we get from them in our health parameters is the most important.*

1.   Are you a Professional or a High level Amateur Athlete?

1.   If your answer is NO, go to the next question.

2.   If your answer is YES, you are a HP5 (High-Performance 5) or a HP4 (High-Performance 4) or a HP3 (High-Performance 3).

Comments: Congratulations! You are at the top of the Chapa Wellness Map. You're an example for all of us; many, many of us have tried and are trying to reach up to that level, so I just want to say that I respect you exceedingly.

Recommendations: You are in a position to lead, so my first recommendation is that you could help us to encourage all your fans and audience all over the world to do Physical Activity; I ask you for that with all my heart. Many are dying today because of this Pandemic. And second is that when you retire, you keep at least your Wellness Level at the Wellness Sweet Spot; we all have seen may retired sports stars with big bellies and more (e.g., Diego Armando Maradona). To finalize with you, I know that you are surrounded with the best experts in sports medicine and that your tests go far beyond the concepts and evaluations of this book, so at this level, you do the tests recommended by your authorities in this field; our goal is to bring people with a Sedentary Life into the WSS, a concept that is well defined in this book. And keep breaking records and looking for the HP5. Good luck!

2. Do you represent your school, university, club, company, yourself, and so on, doing 20 hours or more per week of High Intensity and Medium Intensity Physical Activity or are you a high level amateur Athlete?

1. If you answer is NO, go to the next question.

2. If your answer is YES, you are a HP2 (High-Performance 2) or a HP1 (High-Performance 1).

Comments: Felicitations! You are working hard to be at the top of your Sport or Physical Activity. You are dreaming with the glory; and you are sweating; enduring pain and sacrifices; investing all your resources; being a good representative of your school, university, club, team, company, yourself, and so on; and being resilient overcoming obstacles and adversities to become a professional or a national champion. Keep going for that vision!

Recommendations: The world is dying due to Physical Inactivity; we need your recommendation wherever and whenever you go to invite people to do Wellness. You are an example to follow, and you can make recommendations to many in one direction, going up into the WSS, *where we have Life* through Sports and Physical Activity. And if some have the call to be a full-time athlete, just as you are, great! They can keep moving up in the Chapa Wellness Map, or they can take the direct road to be a High-Performance athlete with the right coaching and direction. And also, whenever you retire, I desire that you at least keep at the WSS. And I hope I see you soon as a professional athlete or as a great amateur athlete or perhaps as a HP5 someday.

3. Do you work as a personal trainer, fitness center instructor, or sports coach?

1. If your answer is NO, go to **question 6**.

2. If your answer is YES, go to the next question.

4. Besides your work as a personal trainer, instructor, or coach, do you compete in any kind of sports events? And you have studies, certificates, or degrees that support you to exercise your work?

1. If your answer is NO, go to the next question.

2. If your answer is YES, you are an F5 (Fitness 5).

Comments: Congratulations! Besides growing in the knowledge of your career, with many studies, and probably you keep studying to give better attention and service to your clients and learning the last training techniques to be actualized in your profession, you keep that competition spirit to win, and to test your abilities and keep improving in your activity preparing for tournaments and sport events is an example for your pupils as well. Great!

Recommendations: You are a full-time Wellness, Fitness, and High-Performance promoter; super! We are in a war against Physical Inactivity. So you are at the top of the Fitness Level, but you are not a full-time Athlete—you are a teacher or personal trainer or coach; you develop kids, teenagers, and adults to be better in sports and, beyond that, *in Life*; you are a leader in this industry. *We need to move the world* so that no more people will die of this Global Pandemic.

5. Do you have studies, certificates, or degrees as personal trainer, coach, or instructor that support you to exercise your work?

1. If your answer is NO, you are an F3 (Fitness 3).

Comments: Felicitations! You have enough knowledge of your Sport or Physical Activity, and people have noticed; you look Fit and athletic, or you are so good in your sport, and people have noticed, that many people have been asking you for tips of your sport or for a diet or how you do a determined exercise or routine or how to execute a stroke, and so on; but you don't have studies. In some countries and companies, you are not allowed to work without capacitation and their certificates, but in others you can, so this is your case; you have learned by experience, and that is very good because you know in practice how to get to the Fitness Level or to play very well a sport, and you have read a lot and attended seminars, but you are not certificated.

Recommendations: It's time that you start to get the right certificates to be a coach for your sport or as an instructor or as a personal trainer, and so on. Whenever you get your first diploma, you will be immediately a F4 (Fitness 4), and this is the heart of this model, Chapa Wellness Map, that as soon as you know your place in it, you can move to a better one and/or to the one where you would like to be at. Another important recommendation is that while working full time and studying, you could soon not have the time and energy to be totally Fit as Fitness is defined in this book. See Matrix 20 × 20 in chapter 8 and **question 7** in the following page; and if this were the case, my advice is that you keep yourself at least in the Wellness Sweet Spot so that it would be fine that you keep the correct levels of BMI and Waist-Hip Ratio and the other recommended tests for this spot. And keep growing!

2.   If your answer is yes, you are an F4 (Fitness 4).

Comments: Congratulations! Capacitation is key for progress, and today more than ever before, knowledge and technology are exploding exponentially; therefore, we must keep up in this race.

Recommendations: Because you may be very busy attending your job schedule and studies, it is probable that you do not now meet the required results of the F1 (Fitness 1) or F2 (Fitness 2) Levels. See **question 7**. So my recommendation is that you keep at least in the WSS; for that, it would be fine if you keep the correct levels of BMI and Waist-Hip Ratio and keep doing the other recommended tests for this level (see Matrix 20 × 20 in chapter 8). You are already a full-time promoter of Physical Activity (you teach, instruct, train, and study); so, again, congratulations for being a warrior against Physical Inactivity. You have the knowledge to help other people to know their Wellness Level with more precision and to *motivate them to move up for a better Life*, so please do it. Keep learning and teaching!

6.   Besides your activity at work***, do you do 10 hours or more per week of intense and moderate physical activity?

1.   If your answer is NO, go to **question 8**.

2.   If your answer is YES, go to the next question.

7.   Is your BMI* below than 24.9 kg/m² and above 18.5 kg/m²? Is your Waist-Hip Ratio** as a man below .89 or as a woman below .85? Is your body perceived by others as Fit? Do you have a High level or a Good level of aerobic condition, strength, aerobic endurance, speed, balance, coordination, flexibility, and power?

1.   If your answer is NO, go to the next question.

2.   If your answer is YES, you are an F2 (Fitness 2) or an F1 (Fitness 1).

Comments: Ok, this is the highest level of physical condition for someone who is not an athlete, very hard to get, very hard to sustain. Felicitations! This is for me the second aspirational goal promoted in the last decades in media related to sports and fitness. To have a good-looking, athletic fit symmetrical body, just behind the goal of being the number one in your sport or activity, requires many years of continuous effort, discipline, knowledge, sacrifices, pain, willpower, character, economic resources, and so on. Many would want to imitate your shape, and with all the new training techniques such as Suspension Training, Functional Training, Core, Balance, Reacting, and so on, you have the *skills to perform* in a very good way in almost any sport, because you have rated yourself as having a High level or a Good level in these skills. The F2 has a High level in these skills, and the F1 has a Good level; that is the only difference. But both are at the Top of Fitness. You can go from this point to wherever you want, and my hope is that you go up in the Chapa Wellness Map.

Recommendation: You are a model for the industry, so you have some weight as a leader to encourage people to Be Active, to Be Well, to Be Alive; we need everybody involved if we want to make a cultural shift, to make a disruptive change in the sports industry current model. We have to be assertive in what we do; we can increase years of people's lives and help them to be of higher quality. So you can remain where you are or become a F3, a F4, or a F5 or maybe go all the way into the High-Performance Levels. Just remember that many people are dying because they haven't discovered the Treasures of Wellness and Fitness; we can help them. And if at some point of your life you can't keep training good enough to keep in this level, look to never go below the Wellness Sweet Spot (see chapter 9).

8. Besides your activity at work***, do you do less than 5 hours per week of moderate and intense physical activity?

1. If your answer is NO, go to **commentary 9.**

2. If your answer is YES, you are a W3 (Wellness 3) or a W2 (Wellness 2) or a W1 (Wellness 1).

Comments: Great! You are ready to move up in the Chapa Wellness Map. This is the sector that we call the *Sedentary Life Style zone*; this is the no-man's-land. This is the place where nobody that loves his or her life wants to be. It is great that now you are aware of the dangers of this Spot; it is great that you have bought this book, that you are reading it, and much better that you are applying it in your life as you have taken this test. Thank you. Please keep reading; it is for your own good.

Recommendations: If you haven't being aware that Physical Inactivity is the fourth cause of death worldwide, please read Chapter 1 of this book. Physical Inactivity is as bad as smoking, and I can say that to quit doing it, I mean *to start to move more and to eat healthier, it could be as difficult as quitting smoking.* We are talking about changing habits, bad habits, and that is hard; to leave the TV control at your side and go out to walk for 40 minutes may be very hard sometimes, but if you want to have a new experience in your life, to know what it is to be free of the risks linked with Physical Inactivity, to soon enjoy the Wellness Sweet Spot (see chapter 9), start right now. Go out and walk! To jump to the upper levels in the Chapa Wellness Map, you just have to do 300 minutes or more per week of Physical Activity (150 of vigorous intensity aerobic Physical Activity), and you will be at least a W4 (Wellness 4), you will be getting away of that Killing Sedentary Lifestyle. Leave this Deadly Sedentary Lifestyle zone that is killing more than 5,000,000 people every year as soon as possible; we are here to help you. You won't regret it! Visit your physician before you start any exercise program. Try to stay away from injuries so that you can have continuity in your Physical Activity for longer periods of time.

9. Commentary: Now, you fall in the category of doing 5 hours or more and less than 10 hours per week of moderate and intense physical activity; therefore, your Wellness Level by default is a W6 (Wellness 6) or a W5 (Wellness 5) or a W4 (Wellness 4), or you could be

already in the Wellness Sweet Spot (W10, W9, W8, or W7), so go to the next question.

10. Is your BMI* below 24.9 kg/m² and above 18.5 kg/m²? Is your Waist-Hip Ratio** as a man below .89 or as a woman below .85? (You just need the correct level of BMI or Waist-Hip Ratio to answer YES; if you have both of them correct, of course it is a YES).

1. If your answer is NO, you are confirmed by the moment as a W6 (Wellness 6) or a W5 (Wellness 5) or a W4 (Wellness 4).

Comments: Great! You are closer than you think to get into the Wellness Sweet Spot. You are in the Better-But-Not-Enough Zone, you are doing more than five hours per week of Physical Activity, but your levels are still a bit out of where they should be, and your diet could keep improving, so do not worry; you are moving in the right direction.

Recommendations: To be smart is now the name of the game. Visit your physician to see if you can increase the intensity of your Physical Activity. You are doing the right amount of recommended time of physical activity, but the quality of time can be improved. If you manage correctly these 300 minutes or more per week, you can increase the amount of intense aerobic physical activity up to 150 minutes from those 300 minutes of moderate physical activity, doing moderate-intensity aerobic physical activity the rest of the time and combining that time with some muscle-strengthening routines two times per week or more, using your body weight, elastic bands, or dumbbells, involving all your muscles groups. For your diet, see a nutritionist. To jump into the initial levels of the Wellness Sweet Spot, you just need your correct body weight, and this will give us the right BMI. The right diet made by an expert will help you to do this as well. Or getting the right Waist-Hip Ratio also can put you in the lower levels of The Wellness Sweet Spot; all this new Physical Activity and your improved diet will help you to reach the correct Ratio.

2. **If your answer is YES, you are in the Wellness Sweet Spot;** you are a W10 (Wellness 10), W9 (Wellness 9), W8 (Wellness 8), or a W7 (Wellness 7).

Comments: Welcome! *You are living the experience!* I have called this zone the promised land of Wellness, for the reason that here is where our physicians recommend us to be, here is where the risks of getting any disease related to physical inactivity have been considerable reduced; it is a physical condition level that is easier to get and sustain for almost anybody compared to the Fitness Level (see map in chapter 9). It is economically more feasible for everybody in the world compared with High-Performance and Fitness levels.

Recommendations: Learn to enjoy this state and the Physical Activity, diet, and mind-set that have brought you here so that you make it part of your lifestyle. I have designed this Spot in a way that if you have arrived up to the W7 level (Wellness 7), you are already in, *but the more your evaluations results get the correct levels, your risks of getting any disease related to Physical Inactivity are reduced more and more*. Great, don't you think? Also, the higher your level in this Wellness Sweet Spot is going to be. In other words, if you do more than five hours of physical activity per week, and you have your BMI within the correct levels, you are a W7 (Wellness 7); but if you have also your Waist-Hip Ratio right, you will probably be a W8 (Wellness 8). But if your Aerobic Condition is also accurate, then you may be a W9 (Wellness 9), and if your Blood Chemistry (cholesterol, triglycerides, and sugar) is in the right levels as well, you are very close to be a W10 (Wellness 10). At this point, the risks of contracting heart disease, diabetes, breast and colon cancers, and other diseases related to Physical Inactivity have been substantially minimized. *Look to the W10 Level (Wellness 10 Level); it is the safest of all.* I have first placed BMI and Waist-Hip Ratio assessments, because they are from my own perspective the easiest to measure, but the order of the evaluations can be in any other way giving the same increases in the Chapa Wellness Map. To finalize, I just want to say that remaining in this Wellness Sweet Spot, you will be having a much better day-to-day life and a more satisfying aging, giving a bite to the sweetest slice of the universe. I am very happy that you are in this level already or that you have arrived here after looking for it for some period of time, if this is not your first assessment using this system. I am working very hard so that the world can reach this level, the Global Sweet Spot, where we can soon have *zero deaths caused due to Physical Inactivity.*

Schön dass Du hier bist! ¡Genial que estás aquí! (Great that you are here!)

As you may have noticed, to answer all these questions, you just need to have the measurements of your weight, height, waist size, and hip size; the rest of the information is available by counting some hours and by responding other questions, which are very easy to answer, and by doing very easy arithmetical operations. Of course, those who are at the Fitness Levels, like coaches, their knowledge of Skill Factors, such as speed, strength, balance, and so on, was easy to know for them. And the athletes of High-Performance have all the specialized staff, knowledge, and resources for these and many more elaborated tests, so they know.

Now that you know your Initial Level, keep it for yourself; it is not to compete with others at the Wellness Levels. *It is a personal tool* that synthetizes important information of your physical condition; you can work with it with your personal trainer, coach, instructor, or physician, but it is for you. It could be used to calculate the levels of Wellness by Physical Activity of the population in general as well; if this could be the case, I hope that you can cooperate. It will be used for good to create better public policy and a better society and world. Thank you!

WHAT ABOUT NUTRITION?

Organic, bio, gluten-free, vegan, vegetarian, and so on, are words that we just do not read in magazines and social media, but these words are associated with products that we see in our supermarkets, groceries, and nutritional stores every day; and I can say that this is great, and it is a trend in developed and developing countries. I see also many people in those stores in sportswear coming or going to a fitness center after buying healthy food. Also, many of them, especially in North America, walk carrying a bottle of pure water to keep the body hydrated, keeping watch on their body weight and sugar intake. On the other hand, in most of the countries that I have visited , the supply of food in the supermarkets and convenience stores is full of simple carbohydrates like sugar, saturated fats, conservatives, and so on, that are related with other diseases as well, and all over we see many fast-food restaurants promoting and selling fried food, hyper-caloric combos, drinks full of sugar and high-calorie desserts, and so on. So in these countries, *the balance is well loaded to the Unhealthy Nutrition Side.*

A high-calorie intake without Physical Activity in most of the population generates overweight and obesity. Let's see some numbers from the OECD (Organisation for Economic Co-operation and Development) report "Obesity Update 2017":

1. More than one in two adults and nearly one in six children are overweight or obese in OECD countries.

2. Adult obesity rates are highest in the United States, Mexico, New Zealand, and Hungary, while they are the lowest in Japan and Korea.

3. Obesity rates are projected to increase further by 2030, and Korea and Switzerland are the countries where obesity rates are projected to increase at a faster pace.

4. Social inequalities in overweight and obesity are strong, especially among women. In about half of the eight countries for which data are available, less-educated women are two to three times more likely to be overweight than those with a higher level of education.

But some actions to correct this situation have already been taken (from the same OECD report):

1. In the last few years, some OECD countries have relied on fiscal policies to increase the price of potentially unhealthy products to encourage a healthier diet, such as Belgium, Chile, Finland, France, Hungary, and Mexico.

2. New developments in communication policies include new easy-to-understand schemes of food labeling, mass media campaigns to increase public awareness, the use of social networks and new technologies for health-promotion campaigns, and reinforced marketing of potentially unhealthy products, especially when directed to children.

In Mexico, where the problem of overweight and obesity is enormous—28.9 percent of its population is obese (February 2018 data)—we see *high-saturated fat, hyper-caloric fast food all over*; we see it in the streets (in small structures made of metal sheet that act like a freestanding small restaurant), out of the subway, at the side of almost every bus stop, outside of schools, and so on. And, you know, this is the food that many people have as a meal; it is a very hard problem to solve for Mexico, because it is cultural and economical, and it is where supply and demand meet due to historical tradition. Strong public policy and education must be applied here.

In the United States, where the problem is bigger, 36.2 percent of its population having a BMI over 30.0, we can see that part of the problem of *unhealthy food* consumption happened many years ago with the appearance of franchises; American adults have 11 percent of their caloric intake from *fast food restaurants* (October 2017 data). These chains have offered new options of healthier meals, with salads as an example, but desserts too high in calories and large beverages with too much sugar are good sellers and profit makers, so new approaches are needed to make a change. And just remember that only 23 percent of Americans meet national exercise guidelines (data from Club Industry Newsbeat, July 5, 2018).

On the other hand, in the most undeveloped countries and locations, we have the situation of poor nutrition, which can lead to a reduced immune system, increased risk of diseases, and weakening of mental and physical development. Therefore, in these places, a very special Physical Activity program should be promoted alongside the right feeding of these populations. I believe it can be done.

We understand *nutrition* as the process of taking food for maintenance, growth, reproduction, health, and disease of an organism. Then, if we know *it is vital for our lives*, why did we give it a very bad interpretation in our culture? Maybe due to that, knowledge is surpassing custom today, but we now have the opportunity to apply all these knowledge to *change the food supply and demand,* for better options of eating, looking for a healthier lifestyle. This will take time, so current business may be able to adapt their product mix and marketing to help grow this trend of healthier nutrition market, to make it the *new standard way of eating.* My hope is that this will happen soon.

So let's close our mouths a bit, open our eyes more, think before we eat, and *move more.*

ARE WE GOING SUSTAINABLE?

Few years ago, when I elaborated the first model of the Chapa Wellness Map, I thought that a book that would be written in the future about the model should be to present a Model for Sports Sustainability, because by promoting more Wellness in Sports, we would have a much better health, and *Health sustains Life;* therefore, it is more sustainable so that, for me, *Sport is at it´s core "pure sustainability"* according to the principles of the Chapa Wellness Map. So the first phrase that I wrote on the model was: A Model for Sports Sustainability. But after thinking deeper, I saw that, of course, the Chapa Wellness Map shows a more sustainable model for sports, but the book was more about presenting A Systematic Approach to Physical Activity, because it was giving the fundaments for the World Classification System of the Levels of Wellness by Physical Activity, among other subjects. So I kept the term "Systematic" for the Book and the concept of "Sustainability" for the Model. But beyond all these concepts, and after talking with family, friends, colleagues, and my publisher, I decided to make the model, system, and book closer to you, the one who needs Physical Activity. It will be more useful to you—you who work to expand your levels of Well-Being—and for those who love sports and look for new ways to understand it today and into the future; therefore, now the book has been becoming: Be Active, Be Well, Be Alive.

Now I want to write a little bit about the need to express the Sustainable Nature of Sports, so the next lines are going to be about that. Let's suppose we are in the Fitness Level F1 or F2. Here we have every biometrical measurement in the correct levels. Now let's think that we live in a heavily polluted city, so after a good workout and a very healthy meal, we just walk in the street to get inside the car. What have we just breathed? Some ozone, nitrogen dioxide, carbon monoxide, methane, lead, mercury, and so on; all these elements increase the risk factors of getting respiratory infections, asthma, heart disease, stroke, lung cancer, among other diseases. Thus, we have found a *new enemy, Polluted Air* (in 2013, air pollution killed 500,000 people in China alone); hence, for a healthier lifestyle, we must also watch what we breathe in. We have analyzed that Physical Activity and Sports are at their core sustainability; hence, we can feed the concepts, services, and techniques with the modern concepts of Sustainable Development; also, let's remember that thousands of years ago, heavy physical activity was in the form of work to survive, *in the middle of nature for our ancestors*, without many of today's polluting elements that modern society has brought. Further, the first sports were also played in the middle of natural environments, such as forests, jungles, rivers, meadows, mountains, deserts, tundra, and so on.

Now, let's go deeper with this analysis. The Sustainable Development Concept, according to the definition given by the Brundtland Commission in October 1987, was described as "development that meets the needs of the present without compromising the ability of future generations to meet their own needs." Generations of the future? (To have generations in the future we need Life, so Life is implicit in Sustainable Development Concepts.) Our kids and teenagers are going to be the sports players of tomorrow and also the people doing Physical Activity. We want them healthy and having at least the same environment as the one that was left to us; therefore, because of the *core, history, and future* of Physical Activity and Sports, *we must develop the Wellness Industry within a sustainable vision.*

In June 2018, while I was chatting via WhatsApp with friends from Chapingo Autonomous University, the agricultural high school in Chapingo, Mexico, where I studied, I recommended them to do daily Physical Activity, and I was writing some actualizations about the First Industrial Revolution of this book (Chapter 2) that day, where we, as humanity, had a workplace shift during that time from open land to factories, and this was harmful for many. The problem remains till now. I commented that the sustainable agricultural activities are, from my perspective, among the best to realize for our Well-Being through history, because we have open fields, plants, oxygen; we move using our muscles; we see the sky, sun, rain, life in general; and so on. While writing to them that working in the family garden is a great Physical Activity, I remembered that the Universidad Autónoma Chapingo developed a concept named "Farmacia Viviente" (Living Pharmacy), which is based on the production of healing plants in the garden of the house, so we have here a great sustainable concept of Holistic Health generation coming out of Mexico to the world, the Wellness Garden, where we can do our Physical Activity while producing natural healing plants.

The world is changing so fast; one of the most important threats for our society today is Global Warming. The ice is melting, the sea level has been rising, rain precipitation has increased across the globe, among other effects. Throughout this book, we have been facing how to tackle the Global Pandemic of Physical Activity. I think that both problems are suffocating us nowadays, but I don't see Physical Activity having the media and international resonance as climate change has. *Zero deaths by Physical Inactivity* should be as important as having well below 2 degrees Celsius as the biggest increase in temperature because of Global Warming, as it was concluded in the Paris Agreement. We need a global agreement in Physical Activity, but in which city? I don't know! Millions of people are dying every year, and much more are not having the Wellness life that they could have.

WHAT CAN WE DO IN THE FOURTH INDUSTRIAL REVOLUTION (INDUSTRY 4.0)?

This Industrial Revolution's new technologies that are merging the digital, physical, and biological worlds are impacting and will keep impacting our society all over the world for many years in a profound manner, with mobile supercomputing, artificial intelligence, smart factories, self-driving cars, genetic editing, intelligent robots, the Internet of Things and for Things, 3D printing, smart cities, nanotechnology, quantum computing, and so on. In the year 2011, at the Hanover Fair in Germany, the term "Industry 4.0" was used for the first time, promoting the computerization of manufacturing, and today we understand Industry 4.0 as a synonym of the Fourth Industrial Revolution.

Some global leaders of the economy comment that we are going to be able to regenerate our natural environment even to the point of restoring the damages that previous industrial revolutions have brought in the past. This is a great positive impact as many others in many sectors of our lives that will come soon. Can you imagine if we could regenerate the good physical condition of our bodies? I believe we can. But we also have to be aware of many perils that we will be facing in the middle of all these changes, such as organizations and governments not being able to adapt, security risks, growing inequality, among other challenges like unemployment, geopolitical fractures, artificial intelligence competing more and more with human intelligence, and so on.

For some futurists, artificial intelligence could be a threat to humanity whenever the singularity point in this matter would be reached, because scientists don't know if robots or super-intelligent computers may become aware of themselves when they become more intelligent than humans in almost everything, so at this point they may make self-decisions that could endanger human existence. For some authors, this is just science fiction, but for others it is a real danger. But we can do Physical Activity, and robots can't; we can enjoy sweating and feel alive running, swimming, or riding a bike, but they can't. Wellness is a human asset that we must enjoy. It is something that makes us more human, stretching our muscles and breathing, doing yoga postures; climbing a wall, defeating our fears to heights; or focusing in our balance while we skate. It is something that demands many skills that our body has, and all those skills are there, ready to be used, enjoyed, and developed.

But here I wonder, what about Physical Activity? Previous industrial revolutions that have given to us modernity with incredible improvements to our society have influenced in an important manner the generation of our current Physical Inactivity Pandemic, so I want to bring now this important global problem stated in this book doing this simple question: Are we going to keep inactive? Or we will be able to utilize this Fourth Industrial Revolution's (Industry 4.0) technologies to turn it around? I can answer to the first question, NO! And to the second, YES! I see that the trend is going that way, going to a turning point soon, as I see more and more important technology companies getting into the Health Smart Solutions, like Intel and Microsoft (I saw their booths with new products at IHRSA 2016 in Orlando, Florida), and I have witnessed in April 2016 leading technological companies from the Silicon Valley such as Facebook, Google, and Apple promoting the use of bicycles (painted with their corporate colors) to go to work and having Fitness and Sports facilities, with the last training techniques, such as functional training, among good exercise equipment and other facilities like sand volleyball courts, football soccer fields, swimming pools, and so on.

So let's think a little closer about all this global trend. Are we going to have Smart Health and Fitness Industry? Or with the Chapa Wellness Map concepts a "Smart Wellness Industry" or a "Wellness 4.0 Industry"? I can answer to this with an overwhelming YES! Fitness equipment in clubs and homes, parks, streets, sport facilities, stairs, bicycles, public spaces, corporate wellness spots, and so on, interconnected with our smartphones and/or wearables to centralize and process that data for the use of an individual, a family, club, gym, fitness studio, office, corporation, institution, government, and so on. So after seeing all this coming, I am certain that to promote an individual, local, state, national, and Global W7 Level (Wellness 7), the Wellness Sweet Spot is an attainable goal, because today and tomorrow, as never before, it will be easier and faster to change our behavior for better habits.

Can you imagine? Using all this technology to change our homes, transport systems, and workplaces to the point that we can have planned Wellness workouts all over to end with this inactivity pandemic, solving the problems as the lack of time because we could do our Physical Activity almost wherever and whenever and having many options of healthy food due to abundant sources of information and education that have changed the supply and demand of our meals. This is our present for many, and it should be the future for all. So—

Let´s be smart!

AND MINDFULNESS?

A very special father, Zovek: Teacher, hero, and legend. I really don't know why I am writing about him until this part of the book. When you have a father who is so extraordinary in many fields, such as extreme performer in athletics, high-risk escape artist, professor of multiple disciplines, and a man of such mental strength that he captivated a complete nation in the end of the 1960s and the beginning of the 1970s, I can write about him at any time with great respect and admiration. Francisco Xavier Chapa Del Bosque, a Mexican born in the city of Torreón, México, in April 13, 1940, was the husband of Josefina, my mother; father of one daughter, Diana, and three sons, Francisco, Orlando, and Zovek, who, among many other feats, realized 17,800 sit-ups in eight uninterrupted hours, giving as a gift from a sponsor a toy to a kid for each sit-up made in live open television; who swam eight consecutive hours with the legs chained; who jumped rope for eight continuous hours in an event for the Red Cross; who stopped the initial movement of 12 motorcycles with dental strength; who developed a training system (Vuelo Sin Escalas) and a physical training camp that was used by the Mexican army; who trained many people in his television presentations, giving them health, exercise, and many other advices for a better living for everybody, to the point that it was named Professor Zovek; who presented many real high-risk escapes, putting his life in true danger, that surpassed those of Houdini (this was the way it was reported by Mexican newspapers and television commentators in those days); and many, many, many more spectacular acts and incredible presentations.

And do you know what was his fundamental skill to do all these feats? Family, friends, fans, critics, and myself believe that it was in the Mind; in his ability to concentrate all his strength toward a very specific point; in his ability to be there, in full awareness, in absolute attention. In our time, we could say that it was in his natural and well-developed ability of Mindfulness. He used to breathe with special yoga techniques before any presentation or marathon to concentrate to the fullest, and meditation was a common practice for him that he often recommended to his pupils to do, and that included his children. In a time when nobody talked about that, he was a visionary many years ahead of the rest.

Unfortunately, when he was just starting to internationalize his spectacular career, just one week before travelling to Japan for a month of presentations hired by the Fuji Telecasting Co. Ltd for being the Incredible of the Incredible, after just two filmed movies of seven planned in an initial contract, and after just three years of his first presentation as *Zovek*, he had an unfortunate accident. He arrived hanging from a rope that was tied to a helicopter going to a presentation, where he died. He was just 31 years old; the entire Mexican nation was in shock on day, which was March 10, 1972. To write about his incredible life, with all his teachings, ideas, philosophy, spectacular feats, mysticism, example, mind, and so on, it is more than good enough material for a complete spectacular biographic book. For many Mexicans, he is a superhero and a legend. On August 30, 2018, the Oscar-winning director, scriptwriter, and producer, Alfonso Cuarón Orozco, presented his last movie, *Roma,* at the International Film Festival of Venice of where he won the *León de oro* (Golden Lion). It is also the name of an important neighborhood in Mexico City (CDMX), where he will present Zovek as a representative character of Mexico in the early 70s. He is definitely an example of *an astonishing case of mind power, a mind to the fullest.*

As a side note: After the death of my father, my mother was who sustained us financially as a physical education teacher. She had learned from my father's ideas and systems, and she did a great job taking her children upward. Now I am writing a book about Physical Activity and want honor both of them with all my heart.

Thank you, Father and Mother!

Tennis Mind Travelling, personal experiences. In chapter 3 of this book, I gave you a brief review of the part of my life when I gave my full time to tennis. Now I want to share with you my mind experiences, looking to concentrate in winning that important break or game or match point. Once, when I was practicing in 1985 in San Antonio, Texas, an American friend of mine gave me *The Inner Game of Tennis*, written by Timothy Gallwey, as a gift, because he knew I was struggling to focus on my match play. "Don't get distracted wandering with the mind in the middle of the pressure while playing the point"—I remember that from many advices that this book gave me. I applied them in many ways as trying to keep totally focused in the tennis ball, to the point of seeing not just the brand and number printed in the ball but also seeing the ball's hairy felt in detail. Sometimes I was so concentrated in the ball that the perception of the speed of the ball changed in a way that the ball seemed to move in slow motion, almost frozen; that was great! Other tips given by the author to increase and develop concentration while playing were to smell the ball when it was hit with the racket, to imagine the trajectory of the ball as lines over the court and net, and to listen to the ball when it was hit by the opponent, when it bounced in the court, and when it was hit by the racket. To see the ball when it bounced on racket strings was a very special experience for me; I have to confess that I didn't see that effect often enough, but when I got into that level of *mind in full attention*, I performed my best shots and played many of my best matches.

In those years, Mindfulness was not a common concept as it is nowadays, but analyzing it in retrospect, I can confirm today that all those experiences and exercises were pure Mindfulness; he also recommended not to judge our shots or strokes execution as good or bad; but with accurate observations and practice, the body will naturally adjust to perform at the best possible level. Well done, Timothy; you are a visionary!

But the most interesting experience that I ever had with my mind while playing Tennis was to imagine flying with the ball that I hit, flying all over the net into my opponent's court. That was funny! imagination and visualization was strengthened doing this. I really like it, and it is very amusing. I have done it when practicing hitting the ball, never in a tournament match. This could be a good Mental Wellness Drill for everybody in any sport that uses a ball. Doing this reminds me when Albert Einstein visualized himself at the age of 16, chasing a beam of light in a thought experiment (Gedankenexperiment); what power of imagination he had! Also, this helped him in the development of the Special Theory of Relativity. Flying with the ball could be a great *Mind Exercise for kids*. We never know if we, instead of getting the next Roger Federer, may be finding the next Albert Einstein. Ups!

Mindfulness. I am not an expert in mindfulness, even though I have been involved in many types of meditations since I was in my mother's womb, because she was deep in yoga and psycho-prophylactic for my birth; also, she practiced yoga and meditation with my father, sister, brother, and me, when I was a baby. I have attended in the past many courses of transcendental meditation; I have been in Buddhist retreats meditating 24 hours with some sleep intervals when I was vegetarian. I also practiced candle meditation, looking for deeper concentration when I was a full-time tennis player. I have done chakra balancing and cleansing meditations, Tibetan bells meditations, praying complete nights while studying theology, binaural beats and isochronic tones meditations, yoga breathing exercises (pranayama), and so on. By the way, my sister, Diana, who is an expert and speaker of Mindfulness, had some talks with me during the days that I wrote this section of the book, and after some question-and-answer sessions, some videos that she shared with me and a book that she lent me, I can conclude that for her, *Mindfulness is full attention* that develops parts of the brain that are related to the Well-Being and Mind Wellness of those who practice it, and that, above all, *gives them Happiness*.

So what is Mindfulness? For many, today's popularity of this practice has been initiated by Jon Kabat Zinn in the 1970s; he defines Mindfulness Meditation as "the awareness that arises from paying attention, on purpose, in the present moment and nonjudgmentally." Mindfulness comes from Pali (that is a native language of the Indian subcontinent) term "Sati" (the psychological or spiritual faculty of awareness or mindfulness). For Bhante Henepola Gunaratana, author of *Mindfulness in Plain English*, this practice has three fundamental activities:

1.   Full Attention reminds us what we are doing.

2.   Full Attention sees things as they are.

3.   Full Attention sees the real nature of all the phenomena.

Among the proven benefits of mindfulness and meditation, the Forbes website published an article on July 14, 2016, titled "6 Scientifically Proven Benefits of Mindfulness and Meditation," which has the following topics covered: (1) Mindfulness Reduces Anxiety, (2) Mindfulness Meditation Reduces Implicit Age and Race Bias, (3) Mindfulness-Based Cognitive Therapy (MBCT) May Prevent and Treat Depression, (4) Increase Body Satisfaction, (5) Mindfulness Meditation Improves Cognition, and (6) Mindfulness Meditation Helps the Brain Reduce Distractions.

Great!

Origin? Many authors point out that the origin is in religious and secular traditions of Hinduism, Buddhism, and yoga so that mindfulness has been practiced for thousands of years. Some leaders of the contemporary movement of mindfulness have had Buddhists teachers, as it is the case of Jon Kabat Zinn, which was introduced in the Philosophy of Buddhism and Meditation when he was a student at the MIT University. Yoga, which has its origins more than 5,000 years ago, has exercises that incorporate awareness of the body, a body-mind practice, as mindfulness does as well; also, full attention to breathing are employed in both disciplines. Thus, we can see that these two activities are very related.

Present? Jon Kabat Zinn founded the Mindfulness-Based Stress Reduction (MBSR) program in 1979 at the University of Massachusetts. From here and after numerous scientific papers on the clinical applications of mindfulness in medicine and health care, and many books written, he has helped to expand the movement of Mindfulness all over the world in many institutions, in the fields of medicine, psychology, business, professional sports, among others. Jon Kabat had Buddhist teachers, and he integrated this knowledge with western science, and right here is where we find the fundaments of the present concept of Mindfulness. Today, the practice of mindfulness has been integrated into the corporate world to improve the condition of the workplace and the Well-Being of their staff, so companies like Apple and institutions like the Mayo Clinic and others have integrated and promoted this practice in different ways. For example, Duke University in Durham, North Carolina, has special gardens to walk in peace among nature and beauty; there is a Quiet Room in Duke Cancer Center, which is used for meditation, where staff, faculty, students, and visitors interested in spiritual health or having stress problems or looking for nurturing compassion or just relaxing can participate. That this prestigious and research-oriented university has these nice facilities to practice Mindfulness speaks of its importance in our world today.

Future? Just to start, by knowing the scientific benefits for the health and lives of the people that Mindfulness practice brings, I will recommend it to everybody whom I will encourage in the future to get into Physical Activity and to anyone who may want to listen, read, watch, and so on, any of my writings or presentations promoting to Move Up in the Chapa Wellness Map. It is worth it! In the Silicon Valley as the most advanced tech hub in the world, we have an idea of what may be happening in the future in other parts of the world as the Fourth Industrial Revolution keeps evolving all over; and here, at the Silicon Valley, we can see that more and more companies, like Salesforce for example, are having massive events yearly to promote Mindfulness. Fighting the growing stress and depression in the US population is one of their main goals, because the people involved in technology businesses are under many Stressful conditions, like pressure for delivery times and strong competition with other companies, that generates long work schedules that affects them mentally.

Chapa Wellness Map and Mindfulness? Practicing Full Attention while doing our daily Physical Activity could help us to know more about our bodies. What routines and exercises give us the best improvements in our physical condition, which ones make us feel better, paying Full Attention while we run, for example, could avoid accidents, such as any injury in our ankles and/or feet for a bad step. Being Mindful while eating or before buying junk food could help us to avoid eating that thing that is going to affect our health; or, even better, to not throw our money in the trash, hurting our economics by buying rubbish. While eating our daily food, by just eating it in Total Awareness could help us to taste it better and to eat less. Chewing it longer and swallowing without anxiety, helping our digestion and getting the most of the moment of eating, and by eating less, we will be controlling our weight better, which is key for our BMI (Body Mass Index). And all these actions will be increasing our abilities to meditate better with all the benefits that this generates. Definitively, all the benefits that Mindfulness can bring into our lives will create a Wellness—a Holistic Wellness—and with the *great gain of Happiness*, which probably is the most important benefit obtained when doing regular Meditation. And we can start right away by just focusing on the act of breathing, for example.

All these elements make Mindfulness a great ally of ours, to live longer and better while staying at the Wellness Sweet Spot (WSS). This makes me very happy as well, knowing that we can have a combination of Health and Happiness, where our bodies and minds are in harmony, because we can live in the present without stress and worries and trusting that physically we have the best convenient condition, at the W10 Level of the WSS, for the reason that we have reduced to the maximum the risks of getting any disease related to Physical Inactivity. So let's relax, meditate, and keep moving more. And yes—

Let's be Happy!

Frustration, a subproduct of the Current Model. The side effect that I am highlighting while comparing the Sports Model Today (Chapter 3) vs Chapa Wellness Map model (Chapter 4) is *frustration,* and this is a psychological factor, in the mind. I am not a psychologist at all, but I think here we have an immense important field of study for the forthcoming years due to the Costs of Physical Activity that we have already recognized and the worldwide Pandemic of Physical Inactivity that we are suffering nowadays, that we must make an end of it soon.

The High-Performance Level all over the media has taken the Sports Industry up to a 1.1 percent of Global GDP (estimated), and I see that the frustration of not attaining our goals, looking to be as good as a professional or as Fit as a model, has brought this inconstancy when people get in a health and fitness center. Just see the percentage of attrition, which has been reduced more because of sales strategies selling complete years to new members above the real conviction of many people doing exercise; or in a sports club program, many people end up abandoning it. Therefore, I have presented the WSS as a possible solution for that problem; deeper studies are required to be done by the specialists in this field so that we would have more precise knowledge in the human behavior to go with the correct marketing programs, keeping more people active for longer periods of time, with the goal of reaching the Global Sweet Spot by 2030.

Some questions that needed answer from a psychology viewpoint are—

If Physical Activity is so good to us, why not do it?
If bad nutrition brings to us many health problems, why do we not eat healthier?
If selling too much sweet drinks, high-caloric desserts, fried food, fat food, and so on, brings too many public health problems, why do companies keep selling them?
If governments have recognized that Physical Inactivity has a very high cost for national budgets, why has going to the roots program to stop this situation not yet been implemented?

It is time to think better; it is time to use our minds.

EPILOGUE

Today, after many years of work in this model and preparing the final details of the book to send it to my publisher in Aachen, Germany, so they can make it a real one, I can conclude that the modernity brought by the industrial revolutions has changed all the aspects of our lives everywhere, but I think the place where it really has transformed us, influencing the lowering of Physical Activity with all the bad effects analyzed through this book, could be found in three main places:

1. In the way we live in our homes.

2. In the way we move in our transportation systems.

3. In the way we work at the workplace.

Therefore, if we want to solve this Global Pandemic of Physical Inactivity, we must go and dig deep to create disruptive ways to change the environment of these three important spaces of our lives. I think that all through the pages of this book, we have revised many ideas that could modify these places for the good of our health; however, in this segment of the book, the epilogue I will present more new ideas in detail that will help to change these spaces so that we can keep supporting the efforts of many actors all over the world, to make the transformations required to return to a physically active planet.

A WELLNESS FINANCIAL BANK?

We want the world in the Global Sweet Spot, meaning zero deaths from physical inactivity, so I have thought of making the transition from the Cost of Physical Inactivity into Investing in the Wellness Industry; shifting from correction to prevention; saving the lives of more than 5,000,000 people yearly and to give to billions of people better quality of life; boosting an industry that has all the potential to grow 3× (three times) just by renewing its model to meet the demands and challenges of this Fourth Industrial Revolution that we are starting to live and to correct the problems that has not been able to solve; improving social integration, increasing race and gender harmony, upgrading public spaces, encouraging people to enjoy nature; and in general an industry that can help to create a better world. Definitively we need disruptive Wellness–oriented financial services; therefore, I am writing this section giving new ideas to initiate the debate and brainstorming to make this happen.

GDP vs GPI. We have seen in the last two decades the increasing attention by economists in sustainability matters, because of climate change, and the world seems to start getting more serious to tackle this problem as we have seen in the Paris Agreement signed in 2016. But the need of a paradigm shift doesn't stop there; the fundamental point of this book is to change the model to a new one, where everybody will win. Octavio, my brother-in-law, who is an expert in economics and investment projects, sent me a very special link, a few days before writing these lines, with a presentation made by the Deutsche Bank in 2006, where a graphic is presented showing that GDP doesn't measure Well-Being as happiness, living conditions (including health and environment), and economic Well-Being (including leisure and nonmarket activity). This link also presents a chart named Alternatives to GDP, where I have found very interesting information for the core of this book:

GPI (Genuine Progress Indicator): Includes income distribution, value of household and volunteer work, and subtracts factors such as the costs of crime and pollution.
UN Human Development Index: Combines GDP, health, life expectancy, and education.
Gross National Happiness: Used by Bhutan.
CIW (Canadian Index of Wellbeing): Proposed; would include health, education, and environmental quality.

In chapter 10, we can find that—

Chapa Wellness Map: Proposed; to consider the National Level of Wellness through Physical Activity as an important measure of the economic development of the nations.

In October 2009, Nobel Prize winner in economics Joseph Stiglitz urges world leaders to drop that obsession with GDP and focus more on broader measures of prosperity.

Chapa Wellness Map Level Online and App Calculator: To make everyone aware of their Level of Wellness by Physical Activity, we need to use all the possible means, and the financial institutions are important players to make this happen, I think. My hope is that soon we can start implementing this idea that I am going to describe in the next few paragraphs, an idea that I have already discussed with some people of the financial sector. In the last section of this book, Special Topics, I have presented how any person can find in no more than eight questions, what is his or her level in the Chapa Wellness Map; now, the next step is to develop altogether with a financial institution a website with an App, with the main purpose of giving to their current clients and prospects the opportunity to know with a calculator how good they are related to physical activity and how far they are from the risks of the diseases related to Physical Inactivity. Not only banks but also insurances companies may like this concept.

For many, investment is all about risks and yields. What could be better than reducing to the maximum the risks of dying by Physical Inactivity (6% of all deaths), with the yields of better and longer lives, including, of course, the economic savings for everybody of being healthy? For this, *we need to put the person in the center* altogether with the Wellness concept as it is defined in the Chapa Wellness Map Model and more specifically the Wellness Sweet Spot, which is the goal for almost 95 percent of the global population as I have calculated to achieve the goal of *zero deaths by physical inactivity.* If many users of the financial services through Internet can notice this opportunity of obtaining their Wellness Level in a friendly, easy, and technological way in less than 3 minutes without any fee, with an innovative Chapa Wellness Map Level Calculator, and they get it, we will start to *defeat our foe, Physical Inactivity.*

But if the users can find financial options to go deeper, to facilitate the purchase operations between suppliers of technology as wearables or healthy food or exercise equipment or health and fitness centers or check-up labs or mindfulness retreats or just finding public Wellness parks, and so on, we will be hitting a homerun from the first pitch, because we can start to connect demand with supply to make the transition from Obesity and Physical Inactivity Costs to Wellness Investments with all its short-, medium-, and long-term yields. Can you visualize this happening?

Remember that we have to recover the good things that the industrial revolutions took from us, without losing all the great things that progress and modernity have brought into our lives; so I really think that having this App and Website inside a financial environment could help us to change the three places that we have to: the Home, the Workplace, and the Transportations Systems. We are talking about Smart Money.

Financing your Wellness Home: I have always wondered why we have a space in the kitchen for the fridge and the stove, why we have an area in the bedroom for the closet, and why we have some space in the bathroom for the shower. We do not have a room designed specifically for the treadmill or the elliptical machine or the stationary bike; why? This is all about creating the Wellness Home; it is not just about buying the last infomercial product for our houses that will end to be used as a coat rack; we are talking about changing a complete environment to make a Wellness Home Center, a place that could invite us to get physically active. The *Chapa Wellness Map Calculator* will give us where the people are and to where they should go, but it can also calculate, according to the user needs and budget, how much they have to invest and in what, and a way to get it financial support to immediately start making the change, just in case they may want to invest in their Well-Being; if not, great! They can find options in the city altogether with this *Calculator* where the public sector has already done and will keep doing the investments to offer those services for free; or places where the private sector has done and will keep doing the same to make it more affordable and better for anybody. So the complete Wellness industry (know before as Sports Industry) will be activating the people all over this way, with the benefits for many that we have already discussed.

Let's keep thinking about this Wellness Home, where to use a scale or a body fat tester won't be intimidating at all; where a spot to do some sit ups will be comfortable; where a stretching system will be mimicked in the middle of the bedroom or garden; where a Wellness Garden where we can produce medicine, ornament, or edible plants while doing Physical Activity will be part of our daily routine; or where we can have a quiet room to meditate with all the family, having love and unity as the foundation; and so on. And with this Chapa Wellness Map Level Calculator Site and App having the banking services supporting and connecting the system: This is the main idea, so let's keep taking a look into the other places that we must correct to end with this Global Pandemic of Physical Inactivity. And because of the priority of this project, of course producers and consumers could obtain special interest rates with the local banks that, in turn, could be supported by many financial international institutions as well, as is the case with the Climate Change International Financial Support that was approved in the Paris Agreement, that has the goal of mobilizing US$100 billion a year by 2020 from developed countries for climate action in developing countries. Can you imagine that the people at the lower levels of the Chapa Wellness Map, *the Sedentary Lifestyle levels, could get zero percent interest rates* in their purchases to get supported? Or that Key Projects and Suppliers could get special credits to finance the implementation of their business models?

Financing your Wellness Workplace: So our home is starting to change, but the corporative world needs to change too; remember that modernity keeps many of us seated in front a screen, using elevators and escalators, among other Physical Inactivity promoters. But beyond using the stairs instead of these two systems, which is a great way to start changing our activity in the workplace, what if the workers who finish the month in the Wellness Sweet Spot, obtained with the Chapa Wellness Map Calculator, would receive a monetary bonus from the human resources Wellness Management area, that could in turn be in partly paid by the insurance companies and that could be immediately deposited in the employees' account right after they have received the confirmation of the Wellness assessment? The bank sponsoring the Wellness Calculator will be in the center of all these operations, *promoting Life*; we are financing the change of the Workplace. Can you imagine many workers counting calories eaten and burned and checking their BMI and Waist-Hip Ratio often and walking more or signing up in the Fitness Center or looking for ways to develop a Corporate Wellness Center inside the company's facilities. With these kinds of actions, we could be digging deep in the heart of today's Sedentary Oriented Corporative World, to make a change. *Banks can be big players* to bring to an end this Global Pandemic of Physical Inactivity; we have the ideas and the technology, so what is missing?

Financing your Wellness Transportation Systems: For those who don't work in their homes, they need to move to the workplace and come back; our inactive kids (80% the kids of the world) need to go to the school, and in general we need to move to go shopping, to visit a friend, or to go to the movies. I have seen in many cities of the world that the spaces for riding a bicycle have been increased and improved. This is awesome! But now I would like to propose that the Chapa Wellness Map Calculator Site and App could have a section encouraging innovation to disrupt the transportations systems of the world as well, by inviting entrepreneurs to design systems that are not just Zero Greenhouse Emission Vehicles but that are also Zero Physical Inactivity Vehicles. What? Yes! We have our old friend in this segment, the bicycle, that was invented by the German Karl von Drais in 1818, and to have an idea of the amount of activity, someone who weighs 77 kg (170 lb) and rides a bike for an hour, moving a distance of 20 km (12.43 miles), will burn approximately 647 calories. Definitively we need this activity in many people's lives.

But, you know, we can design new human-powered transportation systems using the legs and the arms at the same time as an example; or we can adapt many inventions as the standing bike that works as a treadmill, but it has two wheels; or we can improve the materials of covered recumbent bicycles to protect the user from rain, pollution, and people (security); or we can adapt the existing hybrid electric and pedal bicycles so that they can transport more than one person; and so on. Just by combining the possible solutions of these two problems, Climate Change and Physical Inactivity, we could get plenty of financial resources for new innovative companies and city projects to recover our physical mobility, killing two birds with one stone.

And, of course, we still having our most ancient, natural, and, for me, *the most reliable Wellness Activity: Walking!*

WELLNESS ECONOMY WITH A BIGGER SHARE OF THE GLOBAL GDP

In 2012, the total Sports Industry value as a percentage of the Global GDP "Gross Domestic Product" was approximately of 1.1 percent. Now let's think that the Sports Industry Leaders, Governments, International Institutions, and NGOs have agreed that to bring to an end those between 3,300,000 and 6,000,000 deaths in a year, it is a good goal; because besides saving lives that is priceless, it is more economically efficient to prevent than to correct the bad effects of Physical Inactivity, so we all—citizens, families, schools, universities, institutions, companies, governments, NGOs, and so on—must focus on tackling this Global Pandemic. Therefore, let's suppose that the Sports and Physical Activity industry gets 8 percent increase every year of the participation of the total Economic World GDP (6% invested from costs of Physical Inactivity + 2% of expansion effect in the middle W4, W5, and W6 and in the upper Wellness levels W7, W8, W9, and W10); but this increase was given because of the investments in the lower Wellness levels (W1, W2, and W3) population of the Chapa Wellness Map, green initial circles, where all the health problems related to Physical Inactivity come, but we also get a new effect, an expansion effect, because when more people get physically activated, more people move to the higher levels in the Chapa Wellness Map. Therefore, the Fitness Level market will grow too with, let's say, a rate of 1.5 percent yearly as a percentage of the global GDP. The High-Performance Level also suffers the same effect, because more people will want to get involved in this level as the whole market is growing. Let's give it a 0.5 percent increase yearly of the global GDP. So what do we have here?

8% Wellness + 1.5% Fitness + 0.5% High-Performance = 10% Increase as a percentage of the World GDP yearly

If we keep investing this 6 percent in Wellness from the budget of the costs of Physical Inactivity, we are redirecting spending into investment, during 12 years as an example; because of the natural expansion of more people involved in Sports and Physical Activity in the upper levels on the Chapa Wellness Map, we get—

(1.1% Sports and Physical Activity Industry market size of global GDP today) x (10% participation yearly growth)^12 years)=[(1.1 x (1.1)^12] = 3.45% of Global GDP.

(3.45% expected size with New Model in 12 years / 1.1% current size with Old Model= 3.14 times growth as a percentage of the Global GDP)

Or 314 percent growth (3.14 x 100% = 314%) as a percentage of the Global GDP, without considering the growth of the economy that is estimated for the next 12 years in 3 percent yearly (PWC report, February 2015; The World in 2050. Will the shift in global economic power continue?).

Now, let's put it in dollars:

Global GDP 2017 Nominal (World Bank): 80,864 Billion dollars

Sports and Physical Activity Industry Economic Participation (1.1%): 890 Billion dollars (Sports Model Today 2018)

Investing 6% of the Current Economic Participation (890 x .06): 53.4 Billion dollars (Redirecting Spending of the Costs of Physical Inactivity into Wellness investment)

Sports and Physical Activity Industry New Economic Participation with New Wellness: 2,789 Billion dollars

Model (3.45%) (In numbers of 2017, but remember that this new economic participation came after investing 6% of the current economic participation in Wellness during 12 years)

Difference between the Old Model and the New Wellness Model (2,789 – 890) 1,899 Billion dollars

(1.899 trillion dollars growth of this redefined Wellness Industry that is almost the size of the economy of Italy the 9th economy of the world in 2017).

Now let's make the projection for 12 years from 2018 to 2029 with a 3% yearly Global Growth of the GDP nominal.

Global GDP 2029 Nominal (3% accumulated annual growth): 115,293 Billion dollars

Sports and Physical Activity Industry Economic Participation (1.1%): 1,268 Billion dollars (Sports Model Today 2018)

Sports and Physical Activity Industry New Economic Participation with New Wellness: 3,978 Billion dollars

Model (3.45%) (In numbers of 2029, but remember that this new economic participation came after investing 6% of the 2017 economic participation in Wellness during 12 years)

Difference between the Old Model and the New Wellness Model (3,978 – 1,268): 2,710 Billion dollars (2.710 trillion dollars growth of this redefined Wellness industry)

NOTE: I want to make clear that the Concept of Wellness that I am using here is the concept of Wellness by Physical Activity that I have been presenting during this book and doesn't include the elements of other uses of Wellness, such as beauty, cosmetics, spiritual retreats, and so on, and this is not because these are not important (they are very important, and they constitute a huge and a very good industry) but because this model has been designed to solve the Global Pandemic of Physical Inactivity that our Current Model of Sports Industry has not been able to do so.

Therefore, with new resources invested in the Wellness Level, looking to reach the Global Sweet Spot, to reduce to zero deaths due to Physical Inactivity and the Costs related to this problem (investing from the costs, to prevent instead of correcting); what do we get here? This Industry just by attending a global need will be as big as 3.45 percent of the Global Economic GDP by 2032, if we start to count in 2020 for the reason that this book will be printed for the first time in 2019. In other words, a 3× growth will happen; interesting, don´t you think? (In the calculations of the previous paragraph, I did it from 2018 to 2029 because the last data available in July 2018 of the annual world GDP was from 2017, so the first year projected was 2018, but that was just to do some numbers, to present how interesting they are with this model.)

GDP Economic Participation of the Transforming Sports Industry 2018–2029

From 1.1% (2017) to 3.45% (2029) of the Global GDP

AXIS Y (% Global GDP)

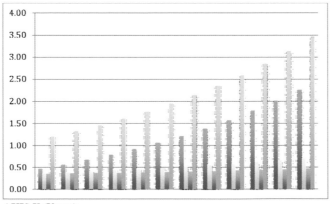

AXIS X (Years)

Blue Column = Total Industry % Global GDP
Red Column = Wellness % Global GDP
Green Column = Fitness % Global GDP
Purple Column = High-Performance % Global GDP
Note: These are just estimated numbers to illustrate the concept and model.

I really have to share this coincidence that I have found. In Mexico, the yearly Cost of Obesity was calculated in 6 billion dollars, and I have estimated roughly that the size of all the Mexican Sports Industry is around those 6 billion dollars (0.56% of the Mexican GDP that was in 2017 of $1,076.914 billions). Funny, don't you think? *An economical resources transfer is clear and necessary here*; can you imagine if Mexico could increase the budget by 6 percent yearly in the Physical Activity and Sports Industry from the Costs of Obesity, with the goal to bring to an end to obesity in 12 years? As we did in the previous paragraphs, giving better life to many people, bringing Mexican national BMI average to correct levels, having *zero deaths by physical inactivity* (Mexico has around 1.7% of the global population, and the global deaths by physical inactivity yearly are of five million (WEF), so 5,000,000 × .017 = 85,000 Mexicans dying every year), having its sports and Wellness Industry growing all over (progress, as you can see, Mexico has an underinvestment in this industry, 0.56% of the Mexican economy compared with the 1.1% participation of this industry in the world, and this underinvestment matches with the Cost of Obesity. Incredible!), with the good effects of lowering crime; increasing national self-esteem; improving public spaces, schools, corporations, and so on; and with more people and kids moving up to the higher levels in the Chapa Wellness Map, the majority into the Wellness Sweet Spot, and others into the Fitness Levels, and strengthening the national High-Performance teams with more people representing with a higher budget to invest.

This is the hearth of the Wellness Economy!

STRATEGIC MANAGEMENT CASE: "WELLNESS/FITNESS/HIGH-PERFORMANCE (AXIS Y)" vs "PRICE POINT $ (AXIS X)"

Now let's do some strategic-management planning. I am going to elaborate a map that on one side, the AXIS Y, is going to have the three levels of physical condition or sports performance proposed by the Chapa Wellness Map: Wellness, Fitness, and High-Performance. On the other AXIS, the X, it is going to have the Price Point Fees ($) of a possible facility, gym, club, park, school and so on. The aim of this graphic is to see where we have to invest, where we have to be innovative, lack of resources being an issue all over the world, and the low price point market segment that has too much need of investment. Here is where the social entrepreneurship has a big chance to participate, and here where the *Low Cost* intersects with the *Wellness segment*, for the reason that in almost all the countries of the world, the lower-income segment are the bigger ones, and as we have seen during this book, the Wellness segment has been largely financially unattended.

First, let's think about the opposite side for a moment to have a general idea of this map (see graph in this chapter). For example, we can visualize the facilities of a Top Professional World-Class Team; what about the Dallas Cowboys? We can imagine the state-of-the-art exercise machines, programs, rehabilitation equipment, sports medicine, analytical software, and so on, which they have to prepare their professional athletes for a High-Performance season in the NFL in the United States representing the city of Dallas in the state of Texas; for sure they have the best. In this region of our graphic, where High-Performance meets the Higher Price Point, it is too high that just the elite professional teams can enjoy. We can find here the facilities of the Manchester United F.C., New York Yankees, Chicago Bulls, FC Bayern München, among other teams.

Second, we are going to look a little bit lower on both AXIS. Let's see the center of the Fitness Level (remember that Wellness has the bigger segment of the population about 95% assumed in this book) intersecting the center of the Price Point ($). What would it be here? I think here we have the average Fitness Club, having many cardiovascular machines, weight machines, free-weight benches, functional training section, group classes rooms, and maybe a swimming pool; here seems that the industry has found a place for growing, where everybody wants to be in, and it is good, as we can see the success and size of the two most important trade shows in the world for this industry—FIBO in Germany and IHRSA in the United States. They are huge and very alive with many new concepts and companies every year and growing. This April 2018, FIBO in Cologne, Germany, had 143,000 visitors and 1,133 exhibitors (11.1% growth compared with 2017), and IHRSA (International Health Racquet and Sportsclub Association) in San Diego, had its 37th world convention and trade show March 2018.

Third, where we have the Wellness Green Circle, as it has been defined in the Chapa Wellness Map, is where we find the great need and opportunity, if we want to make that *Copernican Turn* to change this industry to finish with this Global Pandemic of Physical Inactivity; so if we keep going to lower levels in both AXIS, we will find the point where Wellness matches the Lower Price Point in the market. Here is where the bigger population in the world is, and because in most of the nations there aren't enough financial resources to invest, and not enough buying power of the people in general, here is *the big challenge* for policy makers, politicians, businessmen, researchers, inventors, social entrepreneurs, and so on, to develop low-cost facilities and programs and low price point services and products so that people in this segment may be able to know about and to look to reach the Wellness Sweet Spot (W7-W10). As we have seen before, here is where we have found that *Life meets Sports and Physical Activity* and, with this financial approach, to make it possible for everybody.

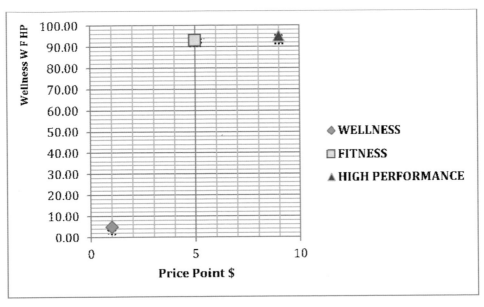

Wellness (W) / Fitness (F) / High-Performance (HP)

VS

Price Point ($)

THE WELLNESS CITY

We are almost concluding this first book of the Chapa Wellness Map series; we need to use all our positive thinking now, all our imagination and creativity, to develop a vision of the Wellness City, a city looking to the WSS (W7–W10) for their inhabitants, *a city able to help them to sustain that level through the years.* What would this Wellness City need for that? I believe that, above all, it will require the involvement of everybody: People, Fitness Instructors, Coaches, Club Managers, Universities, Hospitals, NGOs, Economists, Businessmen, Politicians, among others, to integrate everyone in a proactive way into Physical Activity so that the cultural shift required would happen.

It is not really too complicated, I think, if we notice that it only requires that everyone of us exercise from 50 to 60 minutes five or six times a week; but if we take a look at the surroundings, it can become very hard, first *to teach society* leaders that the people needs to exercise, then teach the people with the media, at schools, in the streets, in parks, and so on, *that Physical Inactivity can kill.* Can you imagine? Signs everywhere as the transit signs indicating that 40 minutes fast walking and 20 jogging and some push-ups and sit-ups five times a week can save your life or that a 40-minute jogging with sit-ups and some yoga postures can help to do that also or that exercise while you walk with your dog can reduce the risk of acquiring diabetes or heart disease; can you imagine? At the side of every public stairs, a sign displaying the amount of calories that would be burned by going up and down for 10 minutes or encouraging the people to do some lunges right there. Can you imagine? A rope with two sizes to measure waist circumference, one for men and one for women, in every public playground or that all the restaurants having a place to do some exercise before eating just as they have a place for the kids to play; can you imagine? All the workplaces with a body fat percentage measurement device to track workers to reach the correct levels or that every fast-food restaurant asking the kids to do 10 push-ups and giving them an exercise Toy after doing it; can you imagine? Universities promoting research to find ways to make all these projects more efficient and more NGOs involved to duplicate the First Wellness City in other cities all over the world; can you imagine? The personal Wellness Data connected with everybody else Wellness Data to have the city Wellness Level on real time; can you imagine? Having in one App all the hours of Physical Activity in a week of the population of a neighborhood, town, or city, and so on. Exciting, right?

This could be a win-win-win project for everybody; current business could invest in new product developments just to change many of the unhealthy food supply existent today, helping to refresh their markets; pharmaceuticals would be able to invest in the development of prevention and in biometry products for Wellness instead of the corrective ones as it is today, also these pharmaceutical companies could sell the products for diseases that are not related to Physical Inactivity, because people will have extra money due to the savings in the sicknesses that they are not getting because they are doing enough Physical Activity, by teaching their clients to invest in prevention rather than in correction of other diseases not related with Sedentary Leifestyles.

And what about the way we move? Our transportation systems, electric cars are coming, many bike circuits are found more and more in many cities all over the world, many universities in Europe are full of bikes, many companies like Facebook, Google, and Apple have many of their employees coming in bikes to their offices; but what can be done to disrupt city transportation for the benefit of Physical Activity? The bicycle is the transport of the future; if people are living not too far from their workplaces, they could go using their legs as motors in new innovative bikes, or walking; remember that thousands of years ago, human legs were the only motors available, so walking and running are great options to recover our active lifestyle. Bikes for polluted cities must be designed, until more bikes will be used there so that pollution would decrease; also, bikes protecting users from robberies are required in some cities, because of violence and insecurity, but here, in the way we all move, we have great opportunities for inventors, and entrepreneurs to create a complete Wellness Mobilization Environment.

Our homes are also a key target to regenerate our sedentary Lifestyle, using our body to generate some energy could be an option. We talked before about the Wellness Garden as well as we have in our houses a special architectonic space for the kitchen and the bedroom, a specific spot for the treadmill of the elliptical machine should be integrated, perhaps in a wall, so that our exercise equipment won't be taking up much space when we are not occupying it. We have to look for video games that make our kids move; it is a funny "coincidence" or a very bad statistical relation that we have around 80 percent of the kids of the world inactive and that the bestselling product of the world in history is a video game console; we need technological and not technological Physical Activity games in our homes. Thousands of years ago, we had daily Heavy Physical Activity in our houses; it is great that with modernity, life became easier at home, but numbers are showing us that we have gone too far. Therefore, for our Wellness City, we need Wellness Homes.

Time goes very fast, but I really think that after implementing some of the concepts stated in this book, somewhere in the world as a neighborhood, a district, or a city will reach soon the Wellness Sweet Spot (W7–W10), setting the bases for the First Wellness City of the world.

HEALTHIER AND HAPPIER AT WORK: FROM W2 TO W10 IN SIX MONTHS

Ok, this is going to be the last theme of this first book, so I want to present an example of how the system could be applied to change any person life, moving her, in this case a woman, from a Sedentary Lifestyle with all the health risks and inconveniences that it has toward the Wellness Sweet Spot. Even though this case is a thought one, it will be very helpful to exemplify how the Chapa Wellness Map could be used in real life, with the people, the ones that we have to bring into this Life Spot, through physical activity, better diet and healthier habits. This is what matters the most!

Let's define the person profile, let's say that she bought this book few months ago, and she liked the ideas and that she got her initial Level of Wellness by Physical Activity as it is explained in the Special Topics Section in the last section and that she obtained a W2 (Wellness 2), that it is almost the lowest possible level so that she contacted us at orlando@chapawellnessmap.info, and she wanted to receive our continuous advice to get away from that harmful Sedentary Lifestyle level to move up into the WSS. She is a 38-year-old woman who works full time as an assistant for a technological company; she is a single mom with one kid and has a dog that she takes to the park one hour on Saturdays and one hour on Sundays. This is the only real Physical Activity that she does during the week, two hours walking with the dog. When she was in high school, she did some track running and volleyball, but nowadays during weekdays, she doesn't have the time to do any Physical Activity because lack of time, too much traffic going and returning from her office, and she loves to be with her 3-year-old kid that her mother helps to look after in the afternoons when the kid has been brought from the kindergarten while she works. At the workplace, most of the time she is seated with just one hour for lunch. In her Chapa Wellness Map assessment, she got a BMI of 29 kg/m^2 and a Waist-Hip Ratio of .92 with a weekly Physical Activity of two hours, which gave her an initial level of W2 (Wellness 2).

First, *we needed to move her from W2 (Wellness 2) to W4 (Wellness 4) level*, instructing her to do at least five hours a week of Physical Activity without taking too much time of her daily activities. So we talked with her, and she accepted the plan; she went to visit her physician to see if everything was all right to start to do more Physical Activity, and after the tests, she was perfect to do more exercise. *The first goal was to walk more*, from two hours to five, so we recommended her to do a 30-minute walk right after her lunch at the office. To make this happen, she talked to her boss to arrive 15 minutes earlier and leave 15 minutes later so that she would be able to take at lunchtime 30 minutes more to do some Wellness Walking around her office's gardens. So how we did start? She was walking at the beginning of her program, 2.5 hours more on weekdays, and we recommended her to walk with her dog 15 minutes more each day, so we were having another 2.5 hours of walking on weekends. So for the first month, we had five hours of low to moderate weekly Physical Activity that wasn't hard for her to assimilate. With these small changes in her lifestyle, she got a new level, and she had already gotten the W4 (Wellness 4). She also visited her nutritionist, who helped to follow a more balanced diet, reducing the intake of fat, sugar, and simple carbohydrates.

Second, we met 30 days later, and we needed to keep moving her up in the levels of the Chapa Wellness Map, to reach the first one of the WSS, the W7 (Wellness 7) level, as our main goal. So we checked her BMI after the first 30 days of this program, and she got 28 kg/m^2 because she reduced her weight from 81.85 kg (180.45 lb) to 79.1 kg (174.39 lb) her height being 1.68 m (5 feet 6 inches); and her Waist-Hip Ratio was also improved to 0.90. *Better but not Enough* scores to be in the Sweet Spot, but she got a W5 (Wellness

5) level. So we talked with her to increase the intensity of her walking and to start to do few minutes of jogging; she was motivated for her improvements and feeling stronger, the clothes started to feel looser; so she accepted. And the new deal for her was that during the weekdays at the office, she must walk at a higher pace those 30 minutes and to walk up the stairs at least five floors and that, during the weekend, in the 1 hour and 15 minutes of walking with the dog to start to do 15 minutes of jogging, 1 hour of walking, and 15 minutes of jogging. These changes needed to be done for 30 days and kept paying attention to the diet; we recommended her to practice some Full Attention while eating to see how she would feel.

Third, then after those 30 days, we contacted each other again to see what had happened, and she said she really wanted to get into the Wellness Sweet Spot zone to rest in the confidence of not having the risk of diseases related to Physical Inactivity so that she learned to do the jogging with her dog, and that was a very funny experience for both. So we calculated her BMI; it was 26.93 kg/m^2 because her weight was 76 kg (167.55 lb) and her Waist-Hip Ratio was 0.88. She said that to do a Mindful Eating helped her to meet her nutritionist's recommendations and that she started to read a book of Mindfulness and that she liked it very much so that she was starting to meditate before going to sleep. So the program was going perfect, and she was doing 300 minutes per week of Physical Activity with a little bit more intensity every time; she was at W6 (Wellness 6) level. So we asked her if she could do more exercise, 15-minute sessions twice a week of strength, combining rubber bands, dumbbells, and body-weight exercises. To this she replied yes. But also we asked her that she needed to increase the Saturday and Sunday jogging with her dog from 15 minutes to 25, reducing 10 minutes of walking with the dog to keep doing 1 hour 15 minutes on Saturday and the same time on Sunday and that, during the 30-minute weekdays walking in her office gardens, instead of five floors, she should do seven floors. She accepted that as well. The right attitude is key for the success of this program. She was doing 5 hours 30 minutes per week of planned Physical Activity.

Fourth, we contacted each other 30 days later, 90 days since the beginning of this journey, and she was feeling much better and getting closer to the WSS; she was a little anxious to know her results. We did our measurements, and she got a BMI of 25.86 kg/m^2 for the reason that her weight was reduced to 73 kg (160.94 lb). Her Waist-Hip Ratio also got better, being 0.86. So 90 days ago when she decided to Move Up in the Chapa Wellness Map Classification System, she was a W2, and after three months of paying attention to the things that really matter for enjoying life better, she had improved four levels. But she remained out of the Wellness Sweet Spoy; she was just 2.7 kg heavier away to get it or two hundredths away in her Waist-Hip Ratio so that she remained in the W6 (Wellness 6) level, very close to the main goal. This time was her initiative to increase the Physical Activity; she said that she would like to buy a bike with a child chair to take her three-year-old son with her to the park on the weekends, 1 hour on Saturday and the same time on Sunday, that she was feeling lighter, stronger, and with much more energy for that, and that she wanted to have her son enjoying the exercise, air, and sun with her. She was totally healthy, so to increase the weekly Physical Activity from 330 minutes to 450 wasn't a problem. Therefore, her new program consisted of 30 minutes of fast walking and ascending seven floors every weekday, 15 minutes of strength training twice a week on weekdays, 1 hour 15 minutes of walking and jogging with her dog (50 minutes walking and 25 minutes jogging) on Saturdays and Sundays, and bike riding with her kid 1 hour on Saturdays and 1 hour on Sundays. So we were all excited with her progress.

Fifth, 120 days since the launching in this adventure, we needed to check if she had gotten into The WSS, so we met her to do the assessments, and we got that she weighed 69.5 kg, giving us a BMI of 24.62 kg/m^2, so after 120 days, and doing more than five hours per week of Physical Activity; with this BMI, she was already there in the Wellness Sweet Spot. We congratulated her, and she was enjoying this moment and felt great. We checked her Waist-Hip Ratio, which was 0.84, so she got it correct. But her running was a little slow to have the recommended aerobic condition, and her blood chemistry and body fat percentage had been planned to be measured for the next month. Therefore, we gave her a W8 (Wellness 8) level. We were all very happy; she told us that she and her mother started to do meditation two to three times per week looking for unity, besides her mother's personal prayers at church. Her Physical Activity program just changed, increasing her jogging time with the dog on weekends from 25 minutes to 40 minutes, and her walking time was reduced from 50 to 35 for Saturdays and Sundays; all the rests remained the same.

Sixth, 150 days after we started with this successful journey, when we met, she told us that she impacted her office in a very positive way toward Physical Activity, that the CEO noticed her changes physically and in attitude so that they decided to create a Wellness Room where they were going to have Zumba classes three times per week and Mindfulness meditations open schedule. And she told us that she received an economic bonus because of her healthier condition; she was reaping more than she had imagined. She already knew how to correctly do the BMI and Waist-Hip Ratio tests, and she got a BMI of 23.74 kg/m^2, and her Waist-Hip Ratio was 0.82. We obtained the results from the laboratory, and her LDL Cholesterol, HDL Cholesterol, and Triglycerides were at the correct levels; so we proceeded to make the Aerobic Condition Test, and she ran the 1.5 miles in 15 minutes, and she got exhausted. She did not pass this time. Therefore, we gave her the W9 (Wellness 9) level. We left the body fat percentage test for the next month and recommended her to increase the intensity of the jogging on Saturdays, reducing the time to 30 minutes with a target Heart Rate of 130 beats per minute and on Sundays to keep her normal jogging pace for 50 minutes.

Seventh, 180 days had passed, six months of this Wellness Pathway, and all the time she showed very good discipline and constancy. To me, those were two key elements for this success story and that she was always paying attention to do not get injured while exercising. She told us that she changed two days of fast walking along with climbing the stairs at her office for two days of Zumba dancing and that her mother was walking with her on weekends to do some activity, so she helped with the dog when she had to do a faster jogging. Her kid looked for her with his bike helmet in his hand on the morning of every weekend, to go bike riding with her; she was ecstatic. So we proceeded to know her test improvements, and yes, they kept getting better. Her BMI was 22.85 kg/m², her Waist-Hip Ratio was 0.80, and her Body Fat Percentage was 25 percent; we didn't make blood chemistry test this time because we did it the month before, and she ran the 1.5 miles in 13 minutes with 30 seconds. So she did it; all her assessments were correct! She got the maximum level of the Wellness Sweet Spot, a 10—the W10 (Wellness 10). She wasn't Nadia Comaneci, but we were all proud of her. *A life had been changed; and if a life can be changed, the whole world can!*

Of course, this imagined story sounds like a Wellness Fairytale, and probably it is; this may be my dream for many people out there. But I just wanted to present to you how this Model, which was classified very academic, scientific and theoretical a year ago, *can be practically applied into our corporate world*, where we have to work hard to finish this Global Pandemic. The next book to be written in these Chapa Wellness Map Books series is going to be named *At the Workplace*, with pure real cases, and I hope we can meet again in that journey. My hope is that you have enjoyed reading all these lines as I have enjoyed writing them; just specifically for this book, I worked 1,500 hours seated in my computer. I did seven international trips during the last three years, and, you know, it has been totally worth it!

Note: For many Instructors and Personal Trainers at the Fitness Studios and Gyms, this method could be slow and boring. Many of them could take their clients into higher levels of Physical Condition faster with less weekly Physical Activity hours, and I believe that they can do it. But unfortunately many people don't have the time and other resources to go to these kinds of facilities, and their workplaces don't have the facilities and programs either. I also believe that one of the reasons many people backslide into Physical Inactivity after going to a Health Club for a short time is because that for them it is harder to keep up with the Physical Activity demands of many club systems, among other reasons. The Attrition percentage and the amount of population not physically active worldwide back me up on this. I really believe that a steady improvement in the levels of Wellness by Physical Activity for the people with a Sedentary Lifestyle is the best way to MOVE them UP to a healthier Lifestyle. Something that for sure will happen is that many people getting active all over will want to receive the specialized training and high-quality services that the Clubs and Gyms all over the world have to offer to them, increasing the numbers of membership with at least the same proportion that we are expecting for the whole New Wellness Industry defined in this book. Therefore:

151,470,000 (Worldwide Club Members 2017) x 3 (Expected Industry growth with New Wellness Model)

=

454,410,000 (Worldwide Club Members 2029)

As a final anecdote, after seven weeks of full-time writing to finish this book, in this second season (the first was two years ago, with 1,000 hours of computer work) and after being strictly following my method, I have to share with you that I just got back to the W9 (Wellness 9) level. I am back into The Wellness Sweet Spot, which, for different reasons, I lost for a few months. But I got today a BMI of 24.86 kg/m^2, and my Waist Circumference was 91 cm (35.83 inches). Two assessments were correct, and I have been running twice a week for an hour in the forest and in the fields of a park near my apartment, and I am running the 1.5 miles test 20 percent faster than the time required for a man of my age; therefore, my aerobic condition is right as well, so I just need to reduce my Waist-Hip Ratio from .94 to .89 to get the recommended result and to do my blood chemistry test again, which was ok the last time, to get the W10 (Wellness 10) level. I believe that at this pace, I could reach it in eight weeks. All this happened today while I was writing the last lines of this book, before sending the complete package to the publisher to get it prepared for printing next year. So I can truthfully tell you that I am already reaping incredible fruits from this project and that I feel very grateful for everything, and I can't stop inviting you to *get by all healthy means inside this boat named the Wellness Sweet Spot.*

Physical Inactivity has won many battles, but it won't win the war.

—Orlando Chapa

GLOSSARY

Aerobic Condition (normally known as cardiovascular fitness, but I would rather say it must be Cardiovascular Wellness): It is the ability of the heart, blood cells, and lungs to supply oxygen-rich blood to the working muscle tissues and the ability of the muscles to use oxygen to produce energy for movement.

Aging: The process of growing older and the appearance of the effects of increasing age.

Athlete (on the Chapa Wellness Map): A person who competes as an amateur or a professional in one or more sports that requires intense physical training (more than 20 hours per week).

Axis: Lines used in a Cartesian coordinated system.

Balance: The ability to move or to remain in a position without losing control or falling.

Blood Chemistry: The determination of the chemical constituents of blood by assay in a clinical laboratory as part of a diagnostic protocol.

Blood Pressure: The pressure exerted by the blood against the walls of the blood vessels, especially the arteries. It varies due to many factors, such as the person's health, age, and physical condition.

Body Composition: The measurement that describes the percentages of fat, bone, water, and muscle in human bodies.

Body Mass Index (BMI): The body mass index (BMI) or Quetelet index is a value obtained from the mass (weight divided by the square of the body height and is expressed in units of kg/m^2).

Bronze Age: The period of time (3,500 BC–1,200 BC) in human history characterized by the use of metals and the development of trade networks.

Classical Antiquity: The period of time (600 BC–AD 500) characterized by the slavery system in Greece and Rome and an economy based on agriculture, trade, and crafts.

Chapa Wellness Map: A new model looking for a systematic approach to physical activity, including sports, labor, and many other activities. That redefines Wellness, Fitness and High-Performance concepts.

Coordination: The ability to move different parts of the body together well or easily.

Corporal Symmetry: The proportion between different parts of the body, creating an aesthetic body.

Cost: Something that is lost, damaged, or given up in order to achieve or get something.

DALY: One DALY can be thought of as one lost year of "healthy" life.

Digital Revolution (Third Industrial Revolution): The period of time (1940–2011) characterized by the change from mechanical and analog electronic technology to digital electronics.

Early Modern Era: The period of time (AD 1,500–AD 1,760) characterized by the great increase in agricultural productivity (Great Britain) and by the high development of mercantilism and international trade.

Economic Development: An increase in living conditions, improvement of the citizen's self-esteem needs, and free and just society.

Elliptical Training: The exercise done in an elliptical trainer that simulates stair climbing, walking, or running, without causing excessive pressure to the joints.

Endurance: The ability or strength to continue or last, especially despite fatigue, stress, or other adverse conditions; stamina.

First Industrial Revolution: The period of time (AD 1,760–AD 1,860) characterized by the transition to new manufacturing processes utilizing waterpower, steam power, machine tools, and so on.

Fit (On the Chapa Wellness Map): The condition of having waist circumference, body mass index, waist-hip ratio, aerobic condition, body symmetry, and blood chemistry (cholesterol and triglycerides) at the correct levels, and good levels of strength, aerobic endurance, speed, balance, coordination, flexibility, and power.

Fitness: Good health, especially good physical condition resulting from exercise and proper nutrition.

Fitness (On the Chapa Wellness Map Model): The level of physical condition where a person is totally Fit. It is located between the Wellness Level and the High-Performance Level. It consists of five levels—from F1 to F5. Here we have the people who, through working-out sessions, right nutrition, discipline, time, knowledge, effort, sweat, money, methodology, and so on, have gotten a body that looks good (and other people notice it) and have enough knowledge of their body, training techniques, diet, exercise equipment, and so on, that many of them become instructors. The main qualitative values of Fitness as I am presenting them are image, shape, discipline, advice, teaching, challenge, profession, perfection, part time, among others.

Fourth Industrial Revolution (Industry 4.0): The current trend of automation and data exchange in manufacturing technologies. Fuses the physical, digital, and biological worlds. From 2011 to ...?

GDP: Gross Domestic Product; it is a monetary measure of the market value of all final goods and services produced in a period of time.

Global W7: The condition where the average on the Classification System Levels of Wellness by Physical Activity of all the nations in the world is on the Wellness Sweet Spot. It is almost as having zero global deaths by Physical Inactivity.

Health: A state of complete physical, mental, and social Well-Being and not merely the absence of disease or infirmity.

High-Performance (On the Sports Model Today): The higher level of sports performance where amateur or professional athletes compete for a prize, representing themselves or their teams, or their nations. It is also used to motivate the sports-industry sales, promotion, and gambling.

High-Performance (On the Chapa Wellness Map): This is the highest level of sports performance, physical activity, or physical condition that is attained after many years of extensive physical training and strict exercise accompanied by a strict diet. The qualitative values of this level are invention, idol, icon, example, champion, records, professional, representation, full time, among others. I have indicated this in the External Circle, on Red Color, right after the Fitness Level.

Industry 4.0: It is synonymous of the Fourth Industrial Revolution and was first called that way in Germany in 2011 at the Hanover Fair.

Iron Age: The period of time (1,200 BC–600 BC) characterized by the use of tools and weapons made of steel and some carbon. In 776 BC, the first Olympic Games were celebrated in Greece.

Jogging: The activity of running at a slow, regular speed, especially as a form of exercise.

Labor: Human activity that provides the goods or services in an economy.

Lifestyle: The typical way of life of an individual, group, or culture.

Map: A diagram or collection of data showing the spatial arrangement or distribution of something over an area.

Mesolithic: The period of time (10,000 BC–7,500 BC) characterized by the gradual domestication of plants and animals. Hunting and fishing to survive along rivers and lakes was a common practice.

Middle Age: The period of time (AD 500–AD 1,500) characterized by the high importance of agriculture and long-distance navigation. Windmills and watermills appeared. Medieval football, horse racing, and fencing were developed in Europe.

Mind: The part of a person that thinks, reasons, feels, and remembers.

NCDs: (Noncommunicable Diseases). Also known as chronic diseases, they are not passed from one person to another. The WHO describes that they tend to be of long duration and are the result of a combination of genetic, physiological, environmental, and behavioral factors.

Neolithic: The period of time (7,500 BC–3,500 BC) characterized by the appearance of division of labor and new crafts, swimming, archery, and wrestling in Libya.

NGO: Nongovernmental Organization; private sector, voluntary (and usually nonprofit and nonsectarian) organization that contributes to, or participates in, cooperation projects, education, training, or other humanitarian, progressive, or watchdog activities.

Nutrition: The substances that you take into your body as food and the way they influence your health.

Paleolithic: The period of time (2,600,000 BC–10,000 BC) characterized by hunting and natural harvesting. Sprinting and wrestling were practiced during this period.

Paradox: Something (such as a situation) that is made up of two opposite things and that seems impossible but is actually true or possible.

Perceived: Past tense of perception (from Latin *perceptio-*, act of perceiving, from *percipere*; a mental image: concept; quick, acute, and intuitive cognition: appreciation; a capacity for comprehension. Synonyms: discernment, insight, wisdom, perceptiveness, perceptivity, sagaciousness, sagacity, sapience).

Physical Activity: Any bodily movement produced by skeletal muscles that require energy expenditure.

Physical Condition: The condition or state of the body or bodily functions.

Physical Inactivity: It is the lack of the required daily Physical Activity bringing many health problems to people and nations. It has been defined as a Global Pandemic with very high economic costs.

Power: The ability of having explosive physical might.

Second Industrial Revolution: The period of time (1860–1940) characterized by the introduction of mass production with the help of electric power and line production. Olympic and professional sports were developed in a global manner.

Sedentary Lifestyle: A type of lifestyle with no or irregular Physical Activity. Sedentary activities include sitting, reading, watching television, playing video games, and using computer for much of the day with little or no vigorous physical exercise.

Strategic Management: A term used to refer to the entire scope of strategic decision-making activity in an organization.

Speed: The ability of being quick.

Stress: A physical, chemical, or emotional factor that causes physical or mental tension and may be a factor in disease causation.

Strength: The ability of being strong; physical power capacity.

Sustainable: Causing little or no damage to the environment and therefore able to continue for a long time.

Sustainable Development: Development that meets the needs of the present without compromising the ability of future generations to meet their own needs.

Sustainable Development Goals (SDGs): The Sustainable Development Goals, otherwise known as the Global Goals, build on the Millennium Development Goals (MDGs), eight antipoverty targets that the world committed to achieving by 2015. The MDGs, adopted in 2000, aimed at an array of issues that included slashing poverty, hunger, disease, and gender inequality and providing access to water and sanitation. Enormous progress has been made on the MDGs, showing the value of a unifying agenda underpinned by goals and targets. Despite this success, the indignity of poverty has not been ended for all.The new SDGs, and the broader sustainability agenda, go much further than the MDGs, addressing the root causes of poverty and the universal need for development that works for all people. UNDP Administrator Helen Clark noted: "This agreement marks an important milestone in putting our world on an inclusive and sustainable course. If we all work together, we have a chance of meeting citizens' aspirations for peace, prosperity, and well-being, and to preserve our planet." The SDGs will now finish the job of the MDGs and ensure that no one is left behind.

Systematic: To present or formulate as a coherent body of ideas or principles.

Third Industrial Revolution (The Digital Revolution): The period of time (1940–2011) characterized by the change from mechanical and electric technology to digital computing. Communication technology expanded greatly. This period marked the beginning of the information technology. This time as never before, less physical activity at the workplace is required to make our everyday living. Women started to appear more often in professional sports.

THE **CHAPA WELLNESS MAP**

Waist Size: Your risk of some health problems is affected by where your body fat is stored, as well as by your weight. Carrying too much fat around your middle (waist) can increase your risk of developing conditions such as heart disease, type 2 diabetes, and cancer. You have a higher risk of health problems if your waist size is more than 91.44 cm (36 inches) if you are a man and more than 80 cm (31.5 inches) if you are a woman.

Wellness: (1) The quality or state of being healthy in body and mind, especially as the result of deliberate effort. (2) An approach to health care that emphasizes preventing illness and prolonging life, as opposed to emphasizing treating diseases.

Wellness (On the Chapa Wellness Map): The level of Physical Activity performance or level of physical condition from the minimal possible level that any person may have up to a point right below where the person is totally Fit. The main values of Wellness presented in this book are feeling good, having good health, relaxation, stress release, weight loss, life-span extension, having fun, socializing, learning, less time required for doing Physical Activity, among others. Here is where most of the world population is, and on this model, I have divided in 10 segments, they being the initial W1 and the final W10. In this level we can find the Wellness Sweet Spot (WSS).

Wellness City: The city having all the following conditions: legal, public policies, infrastructure, knowledge, skilled people, media, and so on, and enough physically active people to reach and sustain an average level of City W7 (Wellness 7) or City Wellness Sweet Spot—in other words, the average of the population of this city is W7 or above, according to the Chapa Wellness Sweet Spot.

Wellness Economy: The share of the total Wellness Industry of the total GDP.

Wellness Garden: A new business model developed by the author, where you get physically activated by producing your own medicinal, ornamental, and edible plants.

Wellness Sweet Spot (WSS): It is the physical condition or sports performance zone or level proposed on the Chapa Wellness Map model, where the risks for Physical Inactivity-related diseases have been diminished in an important manner through moderate- to high-intensity Wellness Physical Activity, and sports and a healthy diet; in this classification system, it is right below the Fitness Level zone and above the Better but not Enough Wellness zone and uses the biometry systems that the new technology is bringing to more people every day in a cheaper and friendly way all over the market. In the Chapa Wellness Map, the WSS is at the W7, W8, W9, and W10 levels that are at the upper levels in the green circle at the center, and for the author it is the promise land of Wellness.

World Classification System of the Levels of Wellness by Physical Activity: The system that will help us after its implementation to classify the countries all over the world to get to know how is the physical condition of its population. It has three main segments, namely, Wellness (W), Fitness (F), and High-Performance (HP), and aims to promote this variable to the point where it is to be considered as an important measure of the economic development of the nations.

World Economic Forum (WEF): An independent nonprofit organization dedicated to improving global economic and social conditions on a global scale. It is well known for its annual meeting held in January in Davos, Switzerland. This is a forum attended by business leaders, political leaders, policy-making leaders, and other leaders to discuss current economic and social issues, ideas, and possible solutions.

World Health Organization (WHO): A specialized agency of the United Nations that is concerned with international public health. It was established on April 7, 1948, and is headquartered in Geneva, Switzerland. The WHO is a member of the United Nations Development Group. Its predecessor, the Health Organization, was an agency of the League of Nations.

World Wellness Network (WWN): The NGO that will be founded by Orlando Chapa Carrillo with the purpose of supporting all the countries that want to receive it to improve their ranking in the World Classification System of the Levels of Wellness by Physical Activity through the generation, sharing and the application of knowledge related to the increase of healthier lifestyles in the population that will reduce the levels of mortality associated with Physical Inactivity. The final goal is to have a Global Wellness Sweet Spot by 2030 and to bring down the number of total deaths to zero.

Zovek: (1) The stage name of the father of the author of this book, who taught him that through Physical Activity, a better life, a better person, a better society, and a better world could come. The best escape artist in all Mexican history. Record man in extreme athletic and dangerous activities. (2) The name of a brother and of a nephew of the author.

REFERENCES

INTRODUCTION

Leonhard, G. (2011). Why data is the new oil and paying with attention is the future of media [Video]. Retrieved from https://youtu.be/kCES2VJoU6g

Schwab, K. (2017). *The fourth industrial revolution.* New York, NY: Crown Business.

United Nations. (1948). Universal declaration of human rights. Retrieved from http://www.un.org/en/universal-declaration-human-rights/

United Nations. (2015). Sustainable development goals. Retrieved from https://www.un.org/sustainabledevelopment/sustainable-development-goals/

CHAPTER 1

Adegoke, B. O., & Oyeyemi, A. L. (2011). Physical inactivity in Nigerian young adults: Prevalence and socio-demographic correlates. *Journal of Physical Activity and Health, 8*(8), 1135–1142. doi:10.1123/jpah.8.8.1135

American Diabetes Association. (2018). Economic costs of diabetes in the U.S. in 2017. *Diabetes Care, 41*(5), 917–928. doi:10.2337/dci18-0007

British Heart Foundation. (2017). Physical inactivity and Sedentary Behaviour Report 2017 [Report]. Retrieved from https://www.bhf.org.uk/publications/statistics/physical-inactivity-report-2017

British Heart Foundation National Centre for Physical Activity and Health. (2014, October 23). Economic costs of physical inactivity [Publication]. Retrieved from http://www.ssehsactive.org.uk/resources-and-publications-item/40/420/index.html

Countries in the world by population. (2018). Retrieved from http://www.worldometers.info/world-population/population-by-country/

Daly, H. E., Cobb, J. B., & Cobb, C. W. (1989). *For the common good: Redirecting the economy toward community, the environment, and a sustainable future.* Boston, MA: Beacon Press.

Databank. (2014). World development indicators. Retrieved from http://databank. worldbank.org/data/reports.aspx?source=2&series=NY.GDP.MKTP.CD&country=

Ding, D., Lawson, K., Kolbe-Alexander, T., Finkelstein, E., Katzmarzyk, P., van Mechelen, W., & Pratt, M. (2016). The economic burden of physical inactivity: A global analysis of major non-communicable diseases. *The Lancet, 388*(10051), 1311–1324.

Fortune 500 2013. (2014, August 13). Retrieved from http://fortune.com/fortune500/ 2013/

García, C. M., & González-Jurado, J. A. (2017). Impacto de la inactividad física en la mortalidad y los costos económicos por defunciones cardiovasculares: evidencia desde Argentina. *Rev Panam Salud Publica, 41*, 92.

Ginsberg, G. M., & Rosenberg, E. (2012). Economic effects of interventions to reduce obesity in Israel. *Israel Journal of Health Policy Research, 1*, 17. doi:10.1186/2045-4015-1-17

Global GDP 2012–2022. (2018). Retrieved from https://www.statista.com/statistics/ 268750/global-gross-domestic-product-gdp/

Hemp, P. (2004). Presenteeism: At work—But out of It. *Harvard Business Review, 82*(10), 49–58.

Inactivity costs the European economy over €80 billion per year. (2015). Retrieved from http://inactivity-time-bomb.nowwemove.com/the-cost-of-physical-inactivity/

Janssen, I. (2012). Health care costs of physical inactivity in Canadian adults. *Applied Physiology, Nutrition, and Metabolism, 37*(4), 803–806. doi:10.1139/h2012-061

Kontsevaya, A., Kalinina, A., & Oganov, R. (2013). Economic burden of cardiovascular diseases in the Russian Federation. *Value in Health Regional Issues, 2*(2), 199–204. doi:10.1016/j.vhri.2013.06.010

Medibank. (2008, October). The cost of physical inactivity. Retrieved from http://www. medibank.com.au/client/documents/pdfs/the_cost_of_physical_inactivity_08.pdf

Mexico GDP—Gross Domestic Product 2016. (2017, October 20). Retrieved from https:// countryeconomy.com/gdp/mexico?year=2016

National Heart Foundation of Australia. (2007, October). Physical activity and depression [Publication]. Retrieved from https://www.heartfoundation.org.au/images/uploads/publications/Physical-activity-and-depression.pdf

Physical exercise improves children's concentration [Web log post]. (n.d.). Retrieved from https://www.kumon.co.uk/blog/physical-exercise-benefits-for-children/

Rovio, S., Kåreholt, I., Helkala, E., Viitanen, M., Winblad, B., Tuomilehto, J., ... Kivipelto, M. (2005). Leisure-time physical activity at midlife and the risk of dementia and Alzheimer's disease. *The Lancet Neurology, 4*(11), 705–711. doi:10.1016/s1474-4422(05)70198-8

Sánchez, V. (2016, March 17). 120 mil mdp al año le cuesta a México la obesidad. Retrieved from http://www.conacytprensa.mx/index.php/ciencia/economia/5827-120-mil-mdp-de-pesos-al-ano-le-cuesta-la-obesidad-a-mexico

South Africa is one of the laziest countries in the world. (2015, September 7). Retrieved from https://businesstech.co.za/news/lifestyle/97711/south-africa-is-one-of-the-laziest-countries-in-the-world/

Third Lancet Series on chronic diseases: Brazil—Key facts. (n.d.). Retrieved from http://www.oecd.org/els/health-systems/thirdlancetseriesonchronicdiseasesbrazil-keyfacts.htm

Uys, M., Bassett, S., Draper, C. E., Micklesfield, L., Monyeki, A., Villiers, A. D., & Lambert, E. V. (2016). Results from South Africa's 2016 report card on physical activity for children and youth. *Journal of Physical Activity and Health, 13*(11 Suppl 2), 265–273. doi:10.1123/jpah.2016-0409

World Health Organization. (2012). Germany physical activity factsheet [Publication]. Retrieved from http://www.euro.who.int/__data/assets/pdf_file/0010/288109/GERMANY-Physical-Activity-Factsheet.pdf?ua=1

World Health Organization. (2014a). Metrics: Disability-Adjusted Life Year (DALY). Retrieved from http://www.who.int/healthinfo/global_burden_disease/metrics_daly/en/

World Health Organization. (2014b). Physical inactivity: A global public health problem. Retrieved from http://www.who.int/dietphysicalactivity/factsheet_inactivity/en/

World Health Organization. (2017). 10 facts on physical activity. Retrieved from http://www.who.int/features/factfiles/physical_activity/en/

Zhang, J. & Chaaban, J. (2013). The economic cost of physical inactivity in China. *Preventive Medicine, 56*(1), 75–78. doi:10.1016/j.ypmed.2012.11.010

CHAPTER 2

Ayres, R. U., & Warr, B. (2005). Accounting for growth: The role of physical work. *Structural Change and Economic Dynamics, 16*(2), 181–209. doi:10.1016/j.strueco.2003.10.003

Bale, J. (2014). Professionals, amateurs and performance: Sports coaching in England, 1789–1914. *Sport in History, 34*(2), 358–360. doi:10.1080/17460263.2014.900275

Beaudreau, B. C. (2006). *The economic consequences of Mr. Keynes: How the second industrial revolution passed Great Britain by.* New York, NY: Iuniverse.

Bell, J. (2017, September 11). The first heart rate monitor invented. Retrieved from https://www.livestrong.com/article/396827-the-first-heart-rate-monitor-invented/

Bod, R. (2013). Early Modern Era: The Unity of the Humanities. *A New History Of The Humanities.* 142–249. Oxford: Oxford University Press. doi: 10.1093/acprof:oso/9780199665211.003.0004

Bojanova, Irena. (2014). The digital revolution: What's on the horizon? *IT Professional, 16*, 8–12. doi:10.1109/MITP.2014.11

Booth, J. (1977). A short history of blood pressure measurement. *Proceedings of the Royal Society of Medicine, 70*(11), 793–799.

Britannica, T. E. (2012, March 12). Friedrich Ludwig Jahn. Retrieved from https://www.britannica.com/biography/Friedrich-Ludwig-Jahn

Britannica, T. E. (2015, December 23). Hand tool. Retrieved from https://www.britannica.com/technology/hand-tool

Britannica, T. E. (2018, March 9). Middle Ages. Retrieved from https://www.britannica.com/event/Middle-Ages

Britannica, T. E. (2018, April 11). Industrial revolution. Definition, facts, & summary. Retrieved from https://www.britannica.com/event/Industrial-Revolution

Britannica, T. E. (2018, May 25). Bronze Age. Retrieved from https://www.britannica.com/event/Bronze-Age

Caswell, A. (2017, February 21). How health club operators should calculate retention rates. Retrieved from http://www.clubindustry.com/trp/how-health-club-operators-should-calculate-retention-rates

Crabbe, T. (2017, April 18). A brief history of working time—And why it's all about attention now. Retrieved from https://inews.co.uk/inews-lifestyle/work/time-no-longer-money-how-to-manage-attention/

Cureton, T. K. (1950). Physical fitness tests of top American athletes. *Journal of School Health, 20*(2), 46–49. doi:10.1111/j.1746-1561.1950.tb01378.x

Davis Cup History. (n.d.). Retrieved from https://www.daviscup.com/en/organisation/davis-cup-history.aspx

De Vries, J. (2009) The limits of globalization in the early modern world. *The Economic History Review, 63*(3), 710–733. Wiley online library. doi:10.1111/j.1468-0289.2009.00497.x

Druzin, R. (2008, September 05). Paralympics traces roots to Second World War. Retrieved from http://www.cbc.ca/sports/olympics-summer/paralympics-traces-roots-to-second-world-war-1.697123

Dunbar, B. (2015, February 19). July 20, 1969: One giant leap for mankind. Retrieved from https://www.nasa.gov/mission_pages/apollo/apollo11.html

Eknoyan, G. (2007). Adolphe Quetelet (1796 1874) the average man and indices of obesity. *Nephrology Dialysis Transplantation, 23*(1), 47–51. doi:10.1093/ndt/gfm517

FIFA. (n.d.a). FIFA World Cup archive. Retrieved from https://www.fifa.com/fifa-tournaments/archive/worldcup/index.html

FIFA. (n.d.b) History of football—The origins. Retrieved from https://www.fifa.com/about-fifa/who-we-are/the-game/index.html

Finkel, J. (2012, May 11). Teddy Roosevelt: The U.S. President that was always rough and ready to throw down. Retrieved from http://www.thepostgame.com/blog/throwback/201210/teddy-roosevelt-athletic-president-fitness-wrestling-boxing

Formula E opens with spectacular crash involving Nick Heidfeld and Nicolas Prost as Lucas di Grassi claims win. (2014, September 13). Retrieved from https://www.telegraph.co.uk/sport/motorsport/11094128/Formula-E-opens-with-spectacular-crash-involving-Nick-Heidfeld-and-Nicolas-Prost-as-Lucas-di-Grassi-claims-win.html

Formula E partners with Prince Albert II of Monaco Foundation. (2014, July 8). Retrieved from http://www.fiaformulae.com/en/news/2014/july/formula-e-partners-with-prince-albert-ii-of-monaco-foundation.aspx

Formula-races-1948. (2015, March 27). Retrieved from https://www.motorsportmagazine.com/archive/article/december-1947/16/formula-races-1948

Gambino, M. (2009). A salute to the wheel. Smithsonian Magazine. [online]. Retrieved from https://www.smithsonianmag.com/science-nature/a-salute-to-the-wheel-31805121/

Gensel, L. (2005). The medical world of Benjamin Franklin. *Journal of the Royal Society of Medicine, 98*(12), 534–538. doi:10.1258/jrsm.98.12.534

Gerd Leonhard's Megashifts. (2015, March 21). Retrieved from https://www.futuristgerd.com/2015/03/21/my-key-ation-trends-right-now-digitization-disintermediation-automation-and-optimization-robotization-and-virtualization-transformation-hellven/

Gorn, E. J., & Goldstein, W. J. (2004). *A brief history of American sports*. Urbana: University of Illinois Press.

Groeneveld, E. (2017, September 29). Paleolithic. Ancient history encyclopedia. Retrieved from https://www.ancient.eu/Paleolithic/

Herlihy, D., & Frassetto, M. (2016, July 19). History of Europe. Britannica. Retrieved from https://www.britannica.com/topic/history-of-Europe/A-maturing-industrial-society#ref311206

History—Ancient history in depth: Bronze Age Britain. (2014). Retrieved from http://www.bbc.co.uk/history/ancient/british_prehistory/bronzeageman_01.shtml

History of fitness. (n.d.). Retrieved from https://healthandfitnesshistory.com/explore-history/history-of-general-fitness/

History of the New York City Marathon. (2017, November 30). Retrieved from https://www.tcsnycmarathon.org/about-the-race/history-of-the-new-york-city-marathon

How did Iron Age people live? (2015). Retrieved from http://www.bbc.co.uk/guides/z8bkwmn

Hull, J. P. (1999). The second industrial revolution: The history of a concept. *Storia Della Storiografia, 36*, 81–90.

IAAF World Championships archive of past events. (n.d.). Retrieved from https://www.iaaf.org/competitions/iaaf-world-championships/history

International Olympic Committee. (n.d.). First Winter Olympics—Chamonix 1924 Winter Olympic Games. Retrieved from https://www.olympic.org/chamonix-1924

International Olympic Committee. (2018, January 19). Ancient Olympic Sports—Running, long jump, discus, pankration. Retrieved from https://www.olympic.org/ancient-olympic-games/the-sports-events

Iron Age: Definition, characteristics, & importance. (n.d.). Retrieved from https://study. com/academy/lesson/iron-age-definition-characteristics-importance.html

Lucas, R. E. (2002). *Lectures on economic growth* (pp. 109–110). Cambridge, MA: Harvard University Press.

Medieval mob football. (n.d.). Retrieved from https://healthandfitnesshistory.com/ ancient-sports/medieval-mob-football/

Méndez, Cristóbal. (n.d.). Retrieved from http://www.museodeldeporte.net/fichas1/ siglo-de-oro/personajes/mendez-cristobal-.html

Middle Age. (n.d.). Retrieved from http://www.dictionary.com/browse/middle-ages

Neolithic Age. (2015). Retrieved from http://www.newworldencyclopedia.org/entry/ Neolithic_Age

Newman, S. (n.d.). Sports in the Middle Ages. Retrieved from http://www.thefinertimes. com/Middle-Ages/sports-in-the-middle-ages.html

Perry, T. P. (2013). Sport in the Early Iron Age and Homeric Epic. In P. Christesen & D. G. Kyle (Eds.), *A Companion to Sport and Spectacle in Greek and Roman Antiquity* (pp. 53–67). Oxford: John Wiley & Sons. doi:10.1002/9781118609965.ch3

Poe, E. (1831) To Helen. The works of Edgar Allan Poe (Lit2Go Edition). Retrieved from http://etc.usf.edu/lit2go/147/the-works-of-edgar-allan-poe/5299/to-helen-1831/

Schoenherr, S. (2004). The digital revolution. Retrieved from http://history.sandiego. edu/gen/recording/digital.html

Schwab, K. (2017). *The fourth industrial revolution*. New York, NY: Crown Business.

Steere, M. (n.d.). Soccer robots being built to beat humans. Retrieved from http://edition. cnn.com/2009/SPORT/football/03/25/robot.football/

Super bowl winners and results. (n.d.). Retrieved from http://www.nfl.com/superbowl/ results/superbowl

Thadeusz, F. (2009, December 24). Alcohol's neolithic origins brewing up a civilization [Web log post]. Retrieved from http://www.spiegel.de/international/zeitgeist/alcohol-s-neolithic-origins-brewing-up-a-civilization-a-668642.html

The Economist. (2012, April 21). The third industrial revolution. Retrieved from https:// www.economist.com/node/21553017

The end of the palaeolithic and the Mesolithic or Epipalaeolithic. (2013). Retrieved from http://www.anthropark.wz.cz/mesolithic.htm

The Mesolithic Period. (n.d.). Retrieved from https://en.natmus.dk/historical-knowledge/denmark/prehistoric-period-until-1050-ad/the-mesolithic-period/

The Old Stone Age (Paleolithic Era). (n.d.). Retrieved from https://www.penfield.edu/webpages/jgiotto/onlinetextbook.cfm?subpage=1525824

The Stone Age: The Mesolithic Period. (2013, August 13). Retrieved from http://www.historyinanhour.com/2013/07/21/the-stone-age-the-mesolithic-period/

Tufft, B. (2014, October 25). This Google exec just smashed Felix Baumgartner's record skydive. Retrieved from https://www.independent.co.uk/news/world/americas/felix-baumgartners-record-breaking-skydive-broken-by-google-executive-alan-eustace-as-he-jumps-from-9817887.html

Ulrich, R. B. (2007). *Roman woodworking* (p. 52). New Haven, CT: Yale University Press.

Violatti, C. (2018, June 04). Neolithic Period. Retrieved from https://www.ancient.eu/Neolithic/

Welch, K. (2007). *The Roman Amphitheatre: From its origins to the Colosseum* (pp. 11–18). Cambridge: Cambridge University Press.

What was life like in the Bronze Age? (2015). Retrieved from http://www.bbc.co.uk/guides/z874kqt

White, M. (2015, April 27). The industrial revolution. Retrieved from https://www.bl.uk/georgian-britain/articles/the-industrial-revolution

Who invented steel: A look at the timeline of steel production. (2017, January 18). Retrieved from https://steelfabservices.com.au/who-invented-steel-a-look-at-the-timeline-of-steel-production/

Wigelsworth, J. R. (2006). *Science and technology in medieval European life* (p. 7). Westport, CT: Greenwood Press.

Wikipedia. (n.d.a). LPGA. Retrieved from https://en.wikipedia.org/wiki/LPGA

Wikipedia. (n.d.b). Sport in Germany. Retrieved from https://en.wikipedia.org/wiki/Sport_in_Germany

Wikipedia. (n.d.c). X Games. Retrieved from https://en.wikipedia.org/wiki/X_Games

World Series Overview. (n.d.). Retrieved from http://mlb.mlb.com/mlb/history/postseason/mlb_ws.jsp?feature=recaps_index

Young, D. C., & Abrahams, H. M. (2018, February 28). Olympic Games. Britannica. Retrieved from https://www.britannica.com/sports/Olympic-Games

CHAPTER 3

7 great reasons why exercise matters. (2016, October 13). Retrieved from https://www. mayoclinic.org/healthy-lifestyle/fitness/in-depth/exercise/art-20048389

25 World's most popular sports (Ranked by 13 factors). (n.d.). Retrieved from https:// www.totalsportek.com/most-popular-sports/

100 most motivational & inspirational sports quotes of all time. (n.d.). Retrieved from http://www.keepinspiring.me/100-most-inspirational-sports-quotes-of-all-time/

Ancient Olympics FAQ 10. (n.d.). Retrieved from http://www.perseus.tufts.edu/ Olympics/faq10.html

Calio, V., Frohlich, T. C., & Hess, A. E. (2014, May 18). 10 best-selling products of all time. Retrieved from https://www.usatoday.com/story/money/business/2014/05/18/24-7-wall-st-the-best-selling-products-of-all-time/9223465/

Fifa corruption crisis: Key questions answered. (2015, December 21). Retrieved from https://www.bbc.com/news/world-europe-32897066

Fitness market facts & stats 2017 [Ideal for business plans]. (2018, January 18). Retrieved from https://www.wellnesscreatives.com/fitness-market-facts-stats-2017/

Fuller, S. (n.d.). Topic: Sports betting—Statistics & facts. Retrieved from https://www. statista.com/topics/1740/sports-betting/

Klein, S. (2017, December 06). LOOK: This is your body on exercise. Retrieved from https://www.huffingtonpost.com.mx/entry/body-on-exercise-what-happens-infographic_n_3838293

Laczo, L. (2017, June 1). How your body changes once you start exercising. Retrieved from https://shapescale.com/blog/fitness/exercising/how-your-body-changes-once-you-start-exercising/

Lance Armstrong receives lifetime ban and disqualification of competitive results for doping violations stemming from his involvement in the United States postal service pro-cycling team doping conspiracy. (2014, March 11). Retrieved from https://www. usada.org/lance-armstrong-receives-lifetime-ban-and-disqualification-of-competitive-results-for-doping-violations-stemming-from-his-involvement-in-the-united-states-postal-service-pro-cycling-team-doping-conspi/

Lance Armstrong stripped of all seven Tour de France wins by UCI—BBC Sport. (2012, October 22). Retrieved from https://www.bbc.com/sport/cycling/20008520

Nike's revenue 2017. Retrieved from https://www.statista.com/statistics/241683/nikes-sales-worldwide-since-2004/

Shazi, N. (2018, February 21). 10 most-watched sport events in the history of television. Retrieved from https://www.huffingtonpost.co.za/2018/02/21/10-most-watched-sport-events-in-the-history-of-television_a_23367211/

Shekhar, A. (2016, August 10). 10 football teams with the best fans in the World. Retrieved from https://www.sportskeeda.com/football/10-football-teams-best-fans-world

Swanson, R. (2017, October 2). Want to clean up college athletics? Pay the players. *The Washington Post.*

Top 25 quotes by Billie Jean King. (of 113). (n.d.). Retrieved from http://www.azquotes.com/author/8027-Billie_Jean_King

CHAPTER 4

Darden, S. (1992, January 31). Super Show expected to draw 88,000 visitors to Atlanta. Retrieved from https://www.upi.com/Archives/1992/01/31/Super-Show-expected-to-draw-88000-visitors-to-Atlanta/2797696834000/

CHAPTER 5

Adidas history. (n.d.). Retrieved from https://www.adidas-group.com/en/group/history/

Marcel Proust—Les 935 citations de Marcel Proust. (n.d.). Retrieved from http://dicocitations.lemonde.fr/auteur/3584/Marcel_Proust.php

World Healt Organization. (2010). *Global recommendations on physical activity for health.* Genève: WHO.

World Healt Organization. (2016, September 01). Constitution of WHO: Principles. Retrieved from http://www.who.int/about/mission/en/

CHAPTER 6

Aldous Huxley quotes. (n.d.). Retrieved from https://www.brainyquote.com/authors/aldous_huxley

Douglas, S., & Nakamura, K. K. (2018, February 26). The world's fastest marathons (and marathoners). Retrieved from https://www.runnersworld.com/races-places/a20823734/these-are-the-worlds-fastest-marathoners-and-marathon-courses/

Perception: Origin and etymology. (n.d.). Retrieved from https://www.merriam-webster.com/dictionary/perception

What is triathlon? (n.d.). Retrieved from https://www.britishtriathlon.org/get-involved/what-is-triathlon

CHAPTER 7

117 Best Benjamin Franklin quotes on health, wealth and wisdom. (n.d.). Retrieved from https://www.sportsfeelgoodstories.com/117-best-benjamin-franklin-quotes/

Global GDP 2012–2022. (2018). Retrieved from https://www.statista.com/statistics/268750/global-gross-domestic-product-gdp/

How big is the sports industry? (2017, November 13). Retrieved from https://medium.com/sportyfi/how-big-is-the-sports-industry-630fba219331

McBride, J. (2018, January 19). The economics of hosting the Olympic Games. Retrieved from https://www.cfr.org/backgrounder/economics-hosting-olympic-games

Sánchez, V. (2016, March 17). 120 mil mdp al año le cuesta a México la obesidad. Retrieved from http://www.conacytprensa.mx/index.php/ciencia/economia/5827-120-mil-mdp-de-pesos-al-ano-le-cuesta-la-obesidad-a-mexico

The World's highest paid athletes 2018. (n.d.). Retrieved from https://www.forbes.com/athletes/#137d7ce455ae

CHAPTER 8

Albert Einstein quotes. (n.d.). Retrieved from https://www.brainyquote.com/quotes/albert_einstein_102390

Blood glucose testing. (n.d.). Retrieved from https://www.diabetes.co.uk/blood-glucose/blood-glucose-testing.html

GCSE Bitesize: Skill related fitness factors. (n.d.). Retrieved from http://www.bbc.co.uk/schools/gcsebitesize/pe/exercise/0_exercise_health_rev3.shtml

Gerd Leonhard's megashifts. (2015, March 21). Retrieved from https://www.futuristgerd.com/2015/03/21/my-key-ation-trends-right-now-digitization-disintermediation-automation-and-optimization-robotization-and-virtualization-transformation-hellven/

Ho-Pham, L. T., Campbell, L. V., & Nguyen, T. V. (2011). More on body fat cutoff points. *Mayo Clinic Proceedings, 86*(6), 584. doi:10.4065/mcp.2011.0097

How much should I weigh for my height and age? (2017, January 05). Retrieved from https://www.medicalnewstoday.com/info/obesity/how-much-should-i-weigh.php

Mayo Clinic. (2017, March 14). How fit are you? See how you measure up. Retrieved from https://www.mayoclinic.org/healthy-lifestyle/fitness/in-depth/fitness/art-20046433

Mayo Clinic. (2018, March 29). Cholesterol test. Retrieved from https://www.mayoclinic.org/tests-procedures/cholesterol-test/about/pac-20384601

National Heart Foundation of Australia. (n.d.). Is my blood pressure normal? Retrieved from https://www.heartfoundation.org.au/your-heart/know-your-risks/blood-pressure/is-my-blood-pressure-normal

Robson, D. (2013, December 17). Symmetry: Why it is important, & how to achieve it! Retrieved from https://www.bodybuilding.com/fun/drobson27.htm

Waist circumference and waist-hip ratio: Report of a WHO expert consultation, Geneva, 11 December 2008. (2011). Geneva: World Health Organization.

CHAPTER 9

C. S. Lewis quotes and sayings—Wise old sayings. (n.d.). Retrieved from http://www.wiseoldsayings.com/authors/c.s.-lewis-quotes/

World hunger, poverty facts, statistics 2016. (n.d.). Retrieved from https://www.worldhunger.org/world-hunger-and-poverty-facts-and-statistics/

CHAPTER 10

The Honorable Thomas Douglas. (1998, January 01). Retrieved from http://www.cdnmedhall.org/inductees/honourable-thomas-douglas

CHAPTER 11

Lavrencic, K., Gosar, A., Allcock, J. B., & Barker, T. M. (n.d.). Slovenia. Retrieved from https://www.britannica.com/place/Slovenia

Luxembourg Declaration on workplace health promotion in the European Union. (n.d.). Retrieved from http://www.enwhp.org/publications.html

The world factbook: México (n.d.). Retrieved from https://www.cia.gov/library/publications/the-world-factbook/geos/mx.html

Thoughts on the business of life. (n.d.). Retrieved from https://www.forbes.com/quotes/430/

World Health Organization. (n.d.) Sustainable development goals. Retrieved from https://www.un.org/sustainabledevelopment/sustainable-development-goals/

CHAPTER 12

World Health Organization. (2018, May 24). The top 10 causes of death. Retrieved from http://www.who.int/news-room/fact-sheets/detail/the-top-10-causes-of-death

SPECIAL TOPICS

Black, J. (2018, April 11). 5 easy ways to practice mindfulness. Retrieved from https://today.duke.edu/2018/04/5-easy-ways-practice-mindfulness

Burgin, T. (2014, April 14). History of Yoga. Retrieved from http://www.yogabasics.com/learn/history-of-yoga/

Chasing a beam of light: Einstein's most famous thought experiment. (n.d.). Retrieved from https://www.pitt.edu/~jdnorton/Goodies/Chasing_the_light/

Cho, J. (2016, July 14). 6 scientifically proven benefits of mindfulness and meditation. Retrieved from https://www.forbes.com/sites/jeenacho/2016/07/14/10-scientifically-proven-benefits-of-mindfulness-and-meditation/#738c3ee663ce

Crespin, C. (2017, November 12). Future of mindfulness in Silicon Valley. Retrieved from https://www.linkedin.com/pulse/future-mindfulness-silicon-valley-colette-crespin

Dillinger, J. (2015, November 02). The most obese countries in the world. Retrieved from https://www.worldatlas.com/articles/29-most-obese-countries-in-the-world.html

Dominic, A. (2018, July 05). Only 23 percent of Americans meet national exercise guidelines. Retrieved from http://www.clubindustry.com/fitness-studies/only-23-percent-americans-meet-national-exercise-guidelines

Global warming effects. (2017, July 14). Retrieved from https://www.nationalgeographic.com/environment/global-warming/global-warming-effects/

Gunaratana, H. (2015). *Mindfulness in plain English*. Somerville, MA: Wisdom Publications.

Health, obesity update. (2017). Retrieved from http://www.oecd.org/health/obesity-update.htm

History of mindfulness: From east to west and from religion to science. (2017, March 14). Retrieved from https://positivepsychologyprogram.com/history-of-mindfulness/

Jon Kabat-Zinn. (2014, June 24). Retrieved from https://www.umassmed.edu/cfm/about-us/people/2-meet-our-faculty/kabat-zinn-profile/

Keeble, B. R. (1988). The Brundtland report: "Our common future." *Medicine and War, 4*(1), 17–25. doi:10.1080/07488008808408783

Mandal, A. (2017, October 30). Obesity and fast food. Retrieved from https://www.news-medical.net/health/Obesity-and-Fast-Food.aspx

Waist circumference and waist-hip ratio: Report of a WHO expert consultation, Geneva, 11 December 2008. (2011). Geneva: World Health Organization.

EPILOGUE

Chapman, G. (2017, March 13). Calories burned biking/cycling calculator. Retrieved from https://caloriesburnedhq.com/calories-burned-biking/

Climate finance roadmap to US$100 billion. (2016, October 17). Retrieved from http://dfat.gov.au/international-relations/themes/climate-change/Pages/climate-finance-roadmap-to-us100-billion.aspx

Final report 2018: Bigger and more international: FIBO a continued success. (2018, April 15). Retrieved from https://www.fibo.com/en/Final-Report-2018-Bigger-and-more-international-FIBO-a-continued-success/59/n386/

Fitness industry trends from IHRSA 2018. (n.d.). Retrieved from https://www.precor.com/en-us/resources/fitness-industry-trends-ihrsa-2018

GDP (current US$). (n.d.). Retrieved from https://data.worldbank.org/indicator/NY.GDP.MKTP.CD

History of the bicycle: A timeline. (n.d.). Retrieved from https://www.brown.edu/Departments/Joukowsky_Institute/courses/13things/7083.html

Mexico GDP—Gross domestic product 2017. (2018, April 25). Retrieved from https://countryeconomy.com/gdp/mexico?year=2017

Price Waterhouse Cooper. (2015). The world in 2050 will the shift in global economic power continue? [Brochure]. UK.

Sánchez, V. (2016, March 17). 120 mil mdp al año le cuesta a México la obesidad. Retrieved from http://www.conacytprensa.mx/index.php/ciencia/economia/5827-120-mil-mdp-de-pesos-al-ano-le-cuesta-la-obesidad-a-mexico

Total population by country 2018. (n.d.). Retrieved from http://worldpopulationreview.com/countries/

Willard, B. (2011, March 08). 5 reasons why a GPI should replace the GDP. Retrieved from https://sustainabilityadvantage.com/2011/03/08/5-reasons-why-a-gpi-should-replace-the-gdp/

PHOTOS

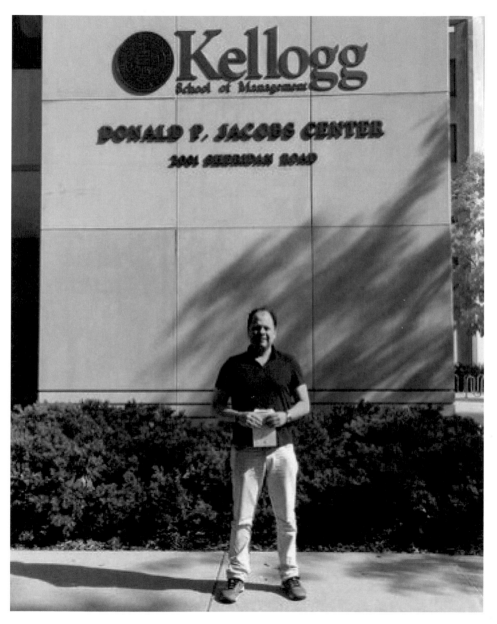

Northwestern University
Promoting the project, 2015

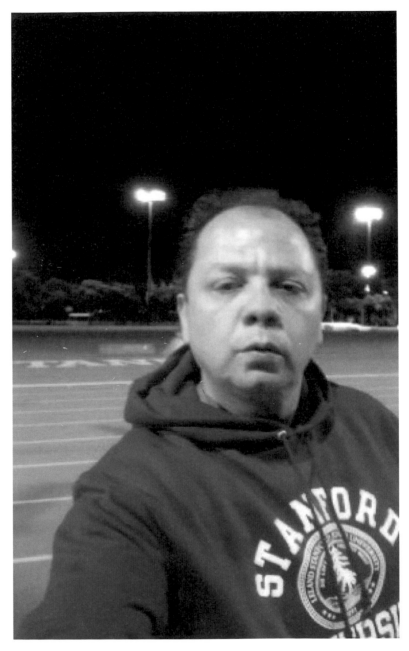

Stanford University
Promoting the project, 2016

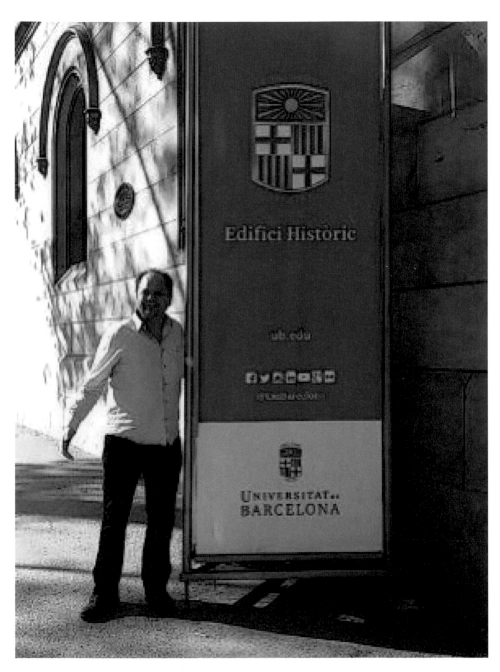

Universitat Barcelona
Promoting the project, 2015

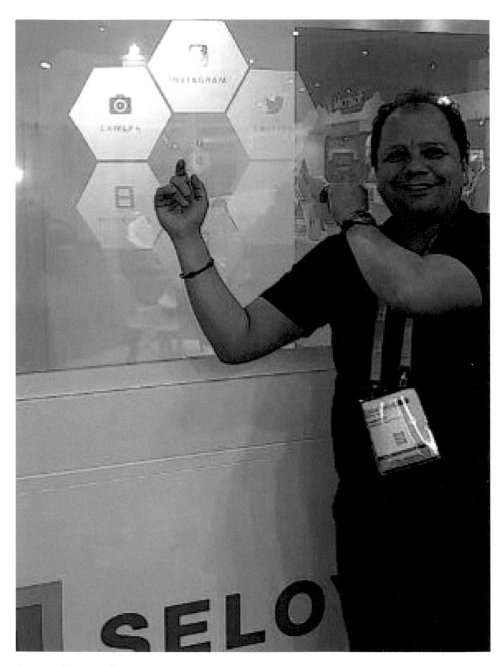

Smart City Barcelona
Promoting the project, 2015

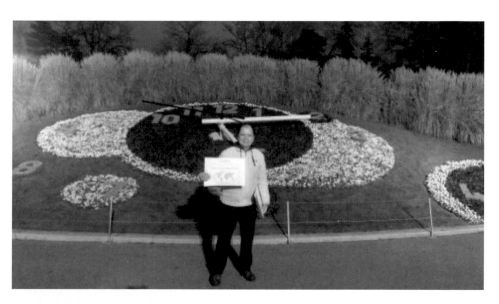

Geneva
Promoting the project, 2015

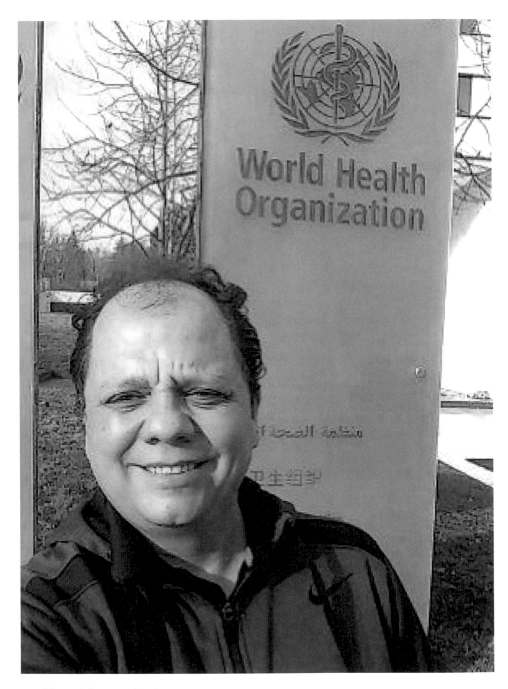

World Health Organization
Switzerland, 2015

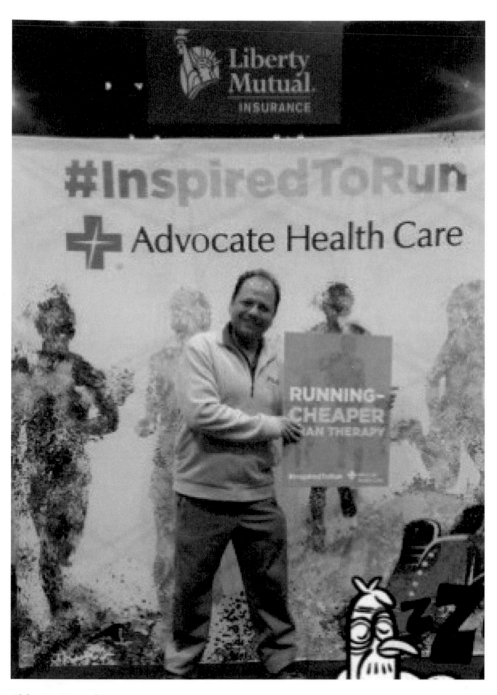

Chicago Marathon
Promoting the project, 2015

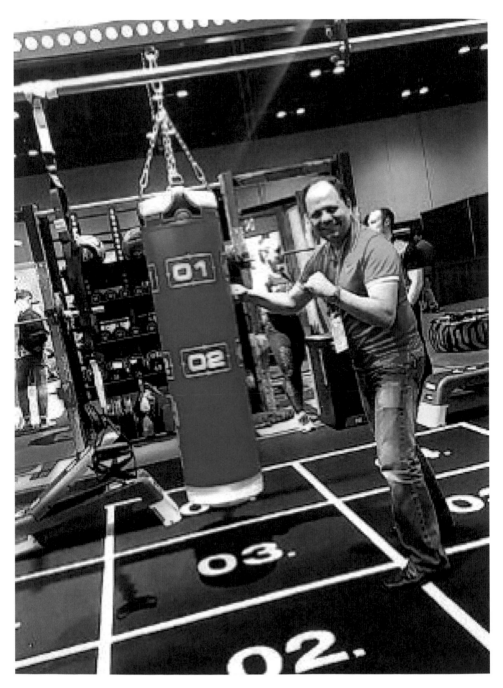

IHRSA, Orlando, 2016

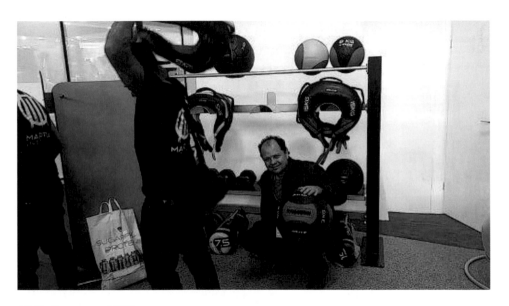

FIBO, Germany, 2016

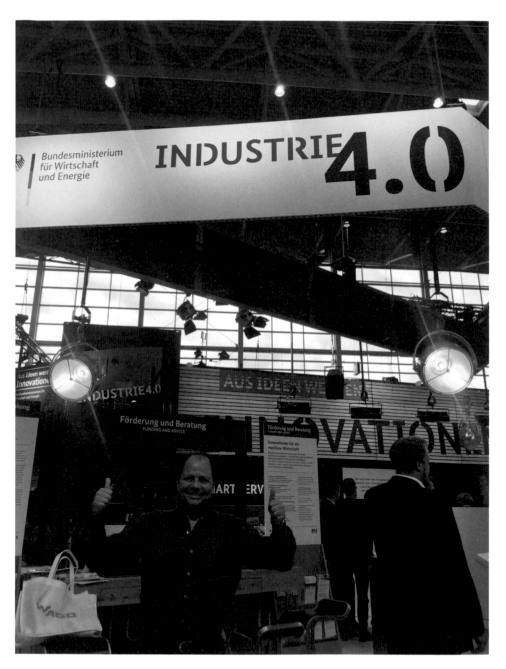

Hanover, 2018

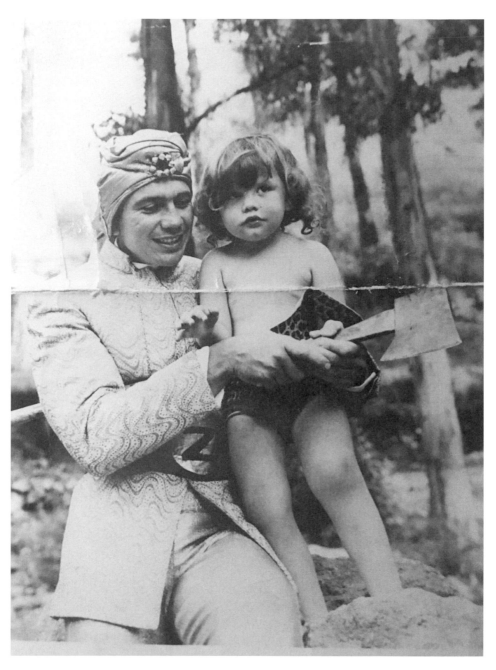

Zovek and his third son, Orlando Chapa Carrillo, 1970

CREDITS

DESIGN & LAYOUT

Cover & interior design: Annika Naas

Layout: Amnet

ILLUSTRATIONS

© Orlando Chapa

PHOTOS

© Orlando Chapa

EDITORIAL

Managing editor: Elizabeth Evans

Copyeditor: Amnet

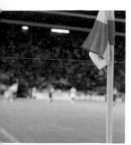

GREAT
FITNESS BOOKS

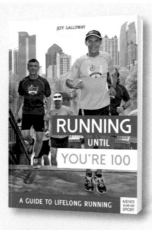

Galloway

Running Until You're 100

A Guide to Lifelong Running

This new edition is the perfect guide for those who want to continue running as they age. The runner can enjoy exercise and enhance life without injury—even until 100!

5th revised edition, 224 p., in color,
69 photos + illus., paperback, 6.5″ x 9.5″
ISBN: 978-1-78255-165-2
$16.95 US

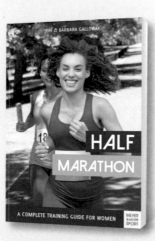

Galloway/Galloway

Half Marathon

A Complete Training Guide for Women

Jeff and Barbara will show you how to select a realistic goal and which workouts are needed to prepare for various running performances. The book deals with issues specific to women as well as universal ones for runners.

2nd revised edition, 216 p., in color,
70 photos + illus., paperback, 6.5″ x 9.5″
ISBN: 978-1-78255-164-5
$18.95 US

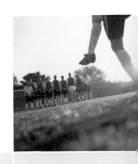
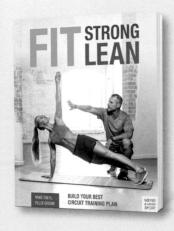
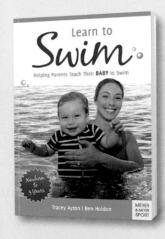

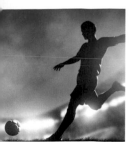
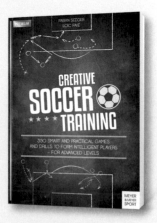
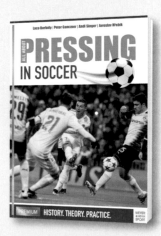

FROM
MEYER & MEYER

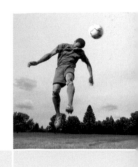

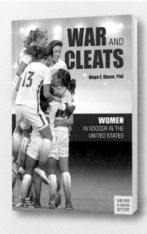

Bhave

War and Cleats

Women in Soccer in the United States

This book offers a contemporary analysis of American women in soccer. Female athletes and coaches are seen as positive cultural icons of gender progress, yet little is known about their everyday experiences in these often male-dominated soccer environments.

200 p., b/w, paperback, 5.5" x 8.5"
ISBN: 978-1-78255-172-0
$19.95 US

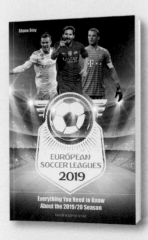

Stay

European Soccer Leagues

Everything You Need to Know About the 2019/20 Season

This book tells readers everything they need to know about Europe's historic soccer leagues. The teams, their histories, their current directions, the key players, coaches, and cities are featured in rich detail.

336 p., b/w, 7 photos + illus.,
paperback, 5.5" x 8.5"
ISBN: 978-1-78255-175-1
$14.95 US